HEALTH EDUCATION

**An Annotated Bibliography on
Lifestyle, Behavior, and Health**

HEALTH EDUCATION

An Annotated Bibliography on
Lifestyle, Behavior, and Health

Marion C. Chafetz
Health Education Foundation
Washington, D.C.

PLENUM PRESS • NEW YORK AND LONDON

ISBN 0-306-40754-X

© 1981 Marion C. Chafetz
Plenum Press is a Division of Plenum Publishing Corporation
233 Spring Street, New York, N.Y. 10013

Printed in the United States of America

To Mosk

ACKNOWLEDGMENTS

I wish to express my appreciation to the following people who worked on the manuscript: Rhonda Vlasak, Cindy Duvall, Gail Dickersin, Jeanne Jefferies, Sylvia Frank, and Barbara Lynch.

My special thanks go to Marie Davies who performed the herculean job of typing the manuscript; to Kaki Maier who helped produce the final product; to Sarah Ober whose special talents and commitment to quality supported my efforts to produce a first-rate bibliography; and to my husband Morris Chafetz whose help and encouragement made the whole thing possible.

CONTENTS

9

FOREWORD

Disease prevention and health promotion have provided an optimistic new look in health policy and practice. The efforts and the products of new ideas, new projects, new programs, new data, new analyses, and new interpretations all have been prodigious. The issue at hand is how to synthesize and summarize this outpouring of new material. In Marion Chafetz' book we have a comprehensive presentation of some of the most tenuous frontiers of disease prevention and health promotion.

The topics covered in this annotated bibliography are the most tenuous topics in the health arena because the ground is shifting so rapidly beneath them, the goals to which they are addressed are so varied and elusive, and the problems they seek to solve are so deeply embedded in our value systems, social structures, and personal privacies. The issues of lifestyle behavior and health do not yield easily to the magic bullets of medicine, nor to the pontification of professors, nor to the mass-manufactured messages of the media. There are as many perspectives on lifestyle and behavior as they relate to health as there are old wives, philosophers, and syndicated doctors. There are as many diets and exercise regimens as there are dietitians and physical educators. Everyone has a prescription for health--providers and consumers alike.

Referring to the tendency of people to believe only their own experience in matters of health, the Food and Drug Administration called it "rampant empiricism." When pitted against the alternative of believing only what professionals say and trying to sort out the multitude of conflicting prescriptions offered by the professionals, FDA might more properly have called it rampant self-preservation of sanity. Moreover, the public has had so many elements of life labelled potentially hazardous to their health that they have begun to despair at the hope of avoiding one risk without running headlong into another. The mass media have delivered the carcinogen of the week with such regularity that there is little left to consume, much less enjoy, if each of these pronouncements were taken seriously.

11

The best hope we have of bringing order out of the
chaos of prescriptions and experiences related to health
promotion is to document as frequently and as thoroughly
as possible the prodigious outpouring of published and
unpublished material describing and analyzing the various
dimensions of health and health behavior. This book offers
a thoughtful sampling of the literature, and the succinct
annotations provide an intelligent documentation of its
contents.

Lawrence W. Green, Dr.P.H.
Director, Office of Health
    Information, Health Promotion
    and Physical Fitness and
    Sports Medicine
Department of Health & Human
    Services

PREFACE

The information explosion of the past two decades has shattered many of our traditional notions of ways to identify, categorize, analyze and synthesize knowledge and has undermined our ability to distinguish the truly new and promising from the old and exhausted. Not that long ago, we saw no problem in mastering the knowledge base of fairly broad subject matters and had little difficulty in separating the wheat from the chaff. More than this, we knew how to translate the accumulated wisdom of an area and its technical foundations into forms comprehensible to the intelligent layman. Knowledge was thought to be finite and standards of excellence and quality straightforwardly applicable.

However we may yearn to return to these comforting notions, the cold facts are that they have been replaced by trends that make processes of "knowledge transfer", "information dissemination", and "diffusion of innovations"-- current buzz phrases for getting information to the public-- all the more difficult. Specialization, an important element in the genesis of the information explosion, has in turn been accelerated to the point that individuals trained in the same basic discipline--whether it be medicine, law, science, education, or other fields--often cannot communicate with one another. Specialists speak in tongues so far removed from everyday English that, more often than not, they cannot articulate their knowledge to outsiders nor relate it to larger questions of concern to the public.

Accompanying this trend is an increasing breakdown in the application of traditional standards of excellence to evaluate new information. At one time, the purveyors of information--the editors and staffs of journals and publishing houses--had the skills and knowledge to serve as watchdogs and gatekeepers. Now the increase in the sheer amount of information as well as its abstruseness has outpaced the number of individuals who possess the needed critical skills and specialized knowledge to evaluate new information. It is not at all uncommon for technically poor or repetitive information to be published. The results of this uneven quality are further complicated by another major contributor to the information explosion:

13

the capacity for high speed electronic transmission of
knowledge, which permits early and widespread distribution
of material. This dissemination often occurs before results have been scrutinized, evaluated, and integrated into
the knowledge base of the specialty from which they proceed.
So much for the gradual accumulation of knowledge tempered
by wisdom, discussion, and reflection.

Faced with a growing volume of highly technical information that is spewed out uncritically by the mass media
it is little wonder that inconsistencies, outright contradictions, and learned argumentation concerning these inconsistencies and contradictions abound--to the increasing
consternation and irritation of a once credulous public
that placed full trust in experts. The blase skepticism
that now characterizes public response to new information
comes as no surprise.

The major institutionalized response to the information explosion has been the development of a new disci-
pline--information science--to cope with the issues,
trends, and problems touched upon above. Basically, the
information scientist is our latter-day librarian. But
unfortunately information science has had the effect of
solidifying and magnifying the problems which it was in
some part intended to solve. The functions of information
science are to identify, acquire, classify, and store information so that it is readily retrievable in forms that
are most useful to those who need it. Offhand, one might
suppose that these functions require specialists who have
more than passing familiarity with the subject matter in-
volved--at least that is what we expect when we go to our
community library or to the local bookstore. Not so, how-
however. Information scientists as a group are proud of
their ability to tackle any body of information to bring
order out of chaos regardless of their knowledge of the
area. Functions, for example, of identification or classification are seen as content free, dependent on guidelines
or thesauri provided by committees of experts drawn from
any given substantive area. With these guidelines and
thesauri, a well-trained clerk can perform the requisite
identification and classification operations--or so the
theory goes. Information scientists are equally proud of
their neutrality with regard to what does or does not go
into an information data base. They eschew all substantive
evaluation processes. Gone is the librarian who orders

books based on an assessment of their quality, contribution
to knowledge, and conceptual permanence. Going is the informative abstract, which summarizes the content and findings of a publication or document, and growing is the indicative abstract, which describes what topics a publication covers but in no way informs the reader how they were
covered. Now, dealing with truly immense quantities of
information obviously requires careful management; but in
its preoccupation with managing the process, information
science has lost much of the value of the art--librarian-
ship--in which it is historically grounded.

Information science, with considerable justification,
relies heavily on computer science, particularly for the
functions of storing and retrieving information. Forward-
looking information scientists point with pride to a time
when books as we know them as well as other print materials
will no longer be necessary and will no longer take up
valuable space in libraries. Instead, that space will be
replaced with computer terminals, microfilm and microfiche
collections, and viewing apparatus. In fact, at least one
university is well on its way to realizing this vision,
computerizing and filming its entire collection.

These uses of information science, of course, fail to
resolve the issues of selectivity, too rapid dissemination
of information, and quality control over intellectual
excellence that were outlined above. In point of fact,
the issues have become more rigidly objectified and institutionalized than before, and with considerable bureau-
cratic reinforcement as schools of information science grow,
supported by public agencies and private organizations.

From the standpoint of the general consumer of technical information, the situation is nowhere worse than in
the health area. The media pander to the unquenchable
thirst of a public anxious for information that will tell
it how to live healthily. This accelerates the widespread
dissemination of early scattered findings, encourages publishers to lower editorial standards, excites scientists
who seek the limelight, and generates seemingly interminable
squabbles over what is indeed healthy and what is indeed
unhealthy. As always, such issues are further beclouded
by economic and social interests that go beyond scientific
fact.

Nowhere is there a greater need for provision of reliable information than in the area of health and behavior.
Which at last brings us to the present work, a work that
aims to take maximum advantage of information science technology while retaining the old values of quality and
relevance. This annotated bibliography, ranging from
aging to yoga, with stops along the way at substance use,
fitness and exercise, bioenergetics, prevention of heart
disease, t'ai chi, among many others, provides lay and
professional reader alike with a guided tour of the best
in the important areas of interrelationship among health,
behavior, and lifestyles. The bibliography is the result
of comprehensive searches of the most recent literature
on the topics. These searches have been conducted by the
highly experienced staff of the Health Education Foundation,
under the able and meticulous leadership of Marion Chafetz,
who brings to the task her many years of background as an
arbiter of health literature and disseminator of health
information. The bibliography represents an extension of
other publication activities carried out by Ms. Chafetz,
including editorship of the HEF Newsletter and Health Fact
Tips, which are published and distributed by the Foundation.

The sprightly, pithy annotations are a welcome break
from the tedium of the indicative abstract. While evalua-
tive and informative, the annotations do not pretend to
exhaustively summarize the content of the original documents
which, in most instances, are full-length books or mono-
graphs. However, each annotation covers the main points
of the author(s) and manages to convey the essential thrust
of the work in the shortest possible manner. The bibliography as a whole should be useful to a wide variety of
users, ranging from the intelligent layman to health practitioners from all fields. It is a first in the HEF Bib-
liographic Series and a suitable complement to Youth,
Alcohol, and Social Policy, the first in the HEF Monograph
Series.

Howard T. Blane, Ph.D.
Professor, School of Education
University of Pittsburgh

INTRODUCTION

If you think good health is all in your mind, then
this bibliography is for you. Designed for both lay and
professional readers, it offers the best selection of
available knowledge about how your attitude toward health--
and your behavior--affects your well-being. All of us
desire good health and long life, and we would like to
remain in good health until we are well advanced in age.

Thanks to dramatic medical advances and an improved
standard of living, Americans now may live much longer than
people did just a few years ago. However, eating too
much or too poorly, smoking too much, or abusing alcohol
can turn these medical gains to ashes.

Of course, such unalterable factors as genetics and
environment are still beyond our control and may touch off
debilitating disease. Nevertheless, three out of five
illnesses result from factors we can control--our eating
habits, our responses to stress, and how much we exercise--
if we choose to.

William Shakespeare seemed to have the answer more
than 400 years ago when he wrote, "The fault lies not in
the stars but in ourselves." Behavioral psychologists
tell us that we are able to change our behavior now more
than ever before.

Millions of people are taking responsibility for their
own health; witness the jogging explosion and record sales
of exercise equipment and self-health literature. Unfortunately, much of this flood of information is conflicting,
inaccurate or unscientific, and separating out scientific
fact from fiction is not easy.

How does one make an intelligent choice? This bibliography cannot make a decision for you, but it certainly
limits the selection to solid, informative works. Each
author is a highly respected authority, an expert in the
field. And all of the books present information about
health that is relevant to the whole person and his or her
environment.

17

You will find chapters with listings on such topics
as alcoholism, drug abuse, fitness and exercise, nutrition,
health education, health in industry, illness and disease
prevention, new areas of health research, and health issues
of special interest to women. That there is no lack of
such information is fortunate; medical knowledge is ex-
panding like an exploding universe. This rapid growth has
drawbacks as well as advantages. Medical costs are sky-
rocketing, making medical services too expensive for many
people to afford, even though they have been encouraged
to believe that good health depends on consumption of
medical services.

But there are benefits as well. One benefit is that
America is increasingly trying to stay healthy. These
efforts are reflected on a national scale by changes in
the food and drug laws, occupational safety and health
rules, a host of environmental regulations and even safer
automobiles. Nonetheless, prevention of illness depends
upon improving personal habits. The obese must decide to
eat less, the smoker to stop smoking, the sedentary to
exercise, the heavy drinker to cut down, and the over-
medicated to rely on the body's own defenses.

Medical science _has_ progressed; the rest is up to you.

                        Marion C. Chafetz
                        Senior Health Editor
                        Health Education Foundation

AGING

The United States has a bad reputation for its attitude toward and treatment of the elderly. Our society
places high value on newness and energy, and low value on
old age and obsolescence. We worship youth, and cultivate
vitality, and cavalierly discard time-worn things. This
attitude is further complicated by our societal over-
emphasis on independence and individuality.

We do our best to make children independent and
responsible. When we admire an "old" person, we often
perceive him or her as "gutsy," a euphemism for independence.

An abundance of articles decry the callous treatment
of our elderly. We like to maintain the myth that we have
treated old people better in the past than we do now. This
myth has been generated and kindled because our response
to old people in the past was different. Few people lived
to be old and those that did were very sturdy. Life expectancy in biblical times was 27 years, and, in 1900, it
had risen to 49.7 years. A female baby born today can
expect to reach age 75 and a male, age 72.

Society as a whole and we as individuals must recognize the increasing ranks of the aged population. In 1900,
only 4 percent of the population was over 65 years. Today,
10 percent is over 65 years, and by 2030, one person in
five or 20 percent of our population will be over 65 years.

Aging populations contain certain universals: the
aged constitute a majority within the population; women
outnumber males, and widows comprise a high proportion of
the older population.

There is a tendency for societies to relegate people
defined as old to sedentary roles; however, people of all
ages require some standard basic needs: the desire to feel
useful and valued and to preserve dignity and self respect.
Modern life demands physical and mental energy. These
fast-paced ways do not accommodate the preconceived mode
of the aged. Ironically, modern technology, which contributed to lengthening the lives of the over-65 group, is

also the source of their problems. Chinese society, which
historically held up its elders as examples of how a society
can respect and integrate its old, is losing status with
the increase in modernization. Formerly, the elderly were
the best source of information for the young. Modern
technological developments and the information explosion
have nullified the need for the elderly to serve as an
information resource.

    Robert Butler, Director of the National Institute
of Aging, said, "If we think back for a moment, we see
that in this century major change has taken place in both
the absolute number and relative proportion of older people.
This change should be regarded as a triumph, for society
has always wanted people to have the opportunity to live
longer."

    World leaders such as Ronald Reagan, Menachem Begin,
Indira Ghandi, and Pope John Paul II to name a few, are
people over 65 who carry heavy official duties while they
lead active private lives. The aged are a great resource
to a society, a vintage blend of information, wisdom,
experience, and perspective. Biological advances have
added years to our lives, and our challenge now is to add
life to our years.

    The selection of books in this chapter broadens know-
ledge about old people and explains the positive aspects
of aging. Many of the books illustrate ways older people
can continue to function as valued members of society and
offer techniques everyone can use to prepare for this
stage of life.

AGING

General

1. Arnold, Oren. THE SECOND HALF OF YOUR LIFE. Harvest
House, Irvine, Calif. 1979.

Humorist, columnist, world traveler, and friendly
neighbor, the author states that the sole purpose of
this book is to alleviate the worry of old age. He
claims straight talk and common sense counsel based on
the vast stores of available knowledge are appreciated
by and helpful to the elderly. He discusses choosing
a place to live, handling money, fostering creativity,
and nurturing faith, as well as other topics.

2. Barrow, Georgia, and Smith, Patricia. AGING, AGEISM
AND SOCIETY. West Publishing, St. Paul, Minn. 1979.

Useful as a high school or college text, this book
focuses upon age and aging in a society that makes
harsh decisions and evaluations about people who are in
the later stages of life. The author attempts to make
the reader aware of a growing "ageist" epidemic and
offers the reader ways to reverse the trend of ageism
in our society.

3. Behnke, John A.; Finch, Caleb B.; and Moment,
Gairdner B., eds. THE BIOLOGY OF AGING. Plenum, New
York. 1978.

4. Binstock, Robert H., and Shanes, Ethel, eds. HANDBOOK
OF AGING AND THE SOCIAL SCIENCES. Van Nostrand
Reinhold, New York. 1979.

5. Burnet, MacFarlane. ENDURANCE OF LIFE. Cambridge
University Press, New York. 1978.

Emphasizing the implications of genetics for human life,
this book delves into the genetics of aging, aging in
mammals, age-associated disease, human diversity, and

21

the decline of the immune system with age. The approach
to aging is both biological and philosophical; the views
are of a retired biologist-pathologist-immunologist now
interested in the aging process.

6. Cape, Ronald D. AGING: ITS COMPLEX MANAGEMENT. Harper
   & Row, New York. 1978.

7. Carlisle, Anthony. AN ESSAY ON THE DISORDERS OF OLD AGE
   AND ON THE MEANS FOR PROLONGING HUMAN LIFE. (Kastenbaum,
   Robert, ed. Aging and Old Age Series.) Arno, New York.
   1979.

8. Carver, Vida, and Liddiard, Penny, eds. AN AGEING
   POPULATION. Holmes & Meier, New York. 1979.

9. Cheyne, George. AN ESSAY OF HEALTH AND LONG LIFE.
   (Kastenbaum, Robert, ed. Aging and Old Age Series.)
   Arno, New York. 1979.

10. Child, Charles M. SENESCENCE AND REJUVENESCENCE.
    (Kastenbaum, Robert, ed. Aging and Old Age Series.)
    Arno, New York. 1979.

11. Cole, Anne P. YESTERDAY'S CHILDREN. Vantage, New York.
    1979.

12. Coleman, Dr. Vernon. EVERYTHING YOU WANTED TO KNOW
    ABOUT AGEING. Gordon-Cremonesi, London, Eng. 1976.

    This useful handbook discusses topics ranging from pre-
    paring for retirement, jobs and hobbies, finances, stay-
    ing healthy, diseases of later life, coping with death,
    and seeking professional care.

13. Comfort, Alex. THE BIOLOGY OF SENESCENCE. Elsevier,
    New York. 1979.

    In this scholarly endeavor, prevailing views of the
    aging process are supported or refuted by an examination
    of evidence from research on animals and man. Dr.
    Comfort believes that the public looks to science to
    understand the mechanisms of senescence. Thus, before
    anyone can devise a means of prolonging individual life,

one must first examine the question in depth from a
biological point of view.

14. Cowdry, Edmund V. PROBLEMS OF AGING: BIOLOGICAL AND
MEDICAL ASPECTS. Arno, New York. 1979.

The information in this volume on aging is highly
clinical and technical; it resembles a medical school
text.

15. Dangott, Lillian, and Kalish, Richard. A TIME TO ENJOY:
THE PLEASURES OF AGING. Prentice-Hall, Englewood
Cliffs, N.J. 1978.

16. DeRopp, Robert S. MAN AGAINST AGING. (Kastenbaum,
Robert, ed. Aging and Old Age Series.) Arno, New York.
1979.

17. Ellison, Jerome. LIFE'S SECOND HALF: THE PLEASURES OF
AGING. Devin, Old Greenwich, Conn. 1978.

Ellison, who wrote this book at age 77, is known to the
reading public as novelist, essayist, critic, reporter,
editor, and educator. He is the founder of the Phoenix
Clubs and president of a nonprofit educational corporation for the study of aging called the Phoenix Society.
Ellison has created this book on aging based mainly on
information in Tibetan Book of the Dead and Schumacker's
Small is Beautiful.

18. Finch, Caleb B., and Hayflick, Leonard. THE HANDBOOK
OF THE BIOLOGY OF AGING. Van Nostrand Reinhold, New
York. 1977.

A number of outstanding experts have contributed to this
exhaustive treatment of the biology of aging. Aging is
considered on the whole-animal level, as well as the
tissue and cellular level. Aging of the skin, separate
organs such as the lung, kidney, and the skeletal-dental
systems are discussed, as well as neoplasia and aging,
the importance of molecular genetics to the subject, and
the evolution of aging throughout the animal kingdom.

19. Fischer, David H. GROWING OLD IN AMERICA. Oxford
    University Press, New York. 1976.

    The author begins with an exaltation of age in early
    America before it became a social problem, and shows
    how devotion to the cult of youth in modern America
    leads to the prevailing attitudes about old age. The
    book offers some interesting thoughts for the future.

20. Fritz, Dorothy B. GROWING OLD IS A FAMILY AFFAIR.
    Knox Press, New York. 1972.

    The author writes frankly and ably from personal ex-
    perience about attitudes toward aging and the aged.
    The book advises the reader to prepare now for later
    years.

21. Hobman, David, ed. THE SOCIAL CHALLENGE OF AGING.
    St. Martin's, New York. 1978.

    This multidisciplinary text is for medical, social, and
    clerical personnel involved in the caring professions,
    as well as for planners and architects whose decisions
    and designs affect the lives of the elderly.

    The book provides a sociological, demographic, and
    cultural background to the role of old people in western
    and eastern societies; it explores the relationship
    which allegedly exists between a number of professional
    disciplines; and considers the structure of an inter-
    disciplinary model.

22. Hornbaker, Alice. PREVENTIVE CARE: EASY EXERCISE
    AGAINST AGING. Sterling, New York. 1974.

23. Huyck, Margaret H. GROWING OLDER: THINGS YOU NEED TO
    KNOW ABOUT AGING. Prentice-Hall, Englewood Cliffs,
    N.J. 1974.

    This book offers an intelligent view of the aging
    process reflecting on current research and theory in
    the field of gerontology. The author offers the aging
    reader a perspective of awareness to deal more effec-
    tively with problems of old age. She presents informa-
    tion to better understand the interaction of such

factors as cultures, economics, social expectations, and norms on the aging phenomenon.

24. Jameson, Thomas. ESSAYS ON THE CHANGES OF THE HUMAN BODY AT ITS DIFFERENT AGES. (Kastenbaum, Robert, ed. Aging and Old Age Series.) Arno, New York. 1979.

25. Jarvik, Lissy F., ed. AGING INTO THE 21ST CENTURY: MIDDLE AGERS TODAY. Halsted Press, New York. 1978.

This anthology is a serious scientific inquiry into all aspects of the aging population, with sections con- tributed by gerontologists, psychiatrists, biochemists, educators, and experts in the field of human development. The question of how cells age, the importance of nutri- tion, aging and intellectual functioning, and societal responses to aging are all treated. This informative book looks to the future and asks: Will senior power become a reality?

26. Kastenbaum, Robert, ed. AGING AND OLD AGE SERIES. Arno, New York. 1979.

27. Kent, Saul. THE LIFE-EXTENSION HANDBOOK: A GUIDE TO BETTER HEALTH, LONGER LIFE AND PHYSICAL IMMORTALITY. Morrow, New York. 1930.

28. Kirk, Clare H. WHEN AGE GROWS YOUNG. (Kastenbaum, Robert, ed. Aging and Old Age Series.) Arno, New York. 1979.

29. Kleemeier, Robert W. AGING AND LEISURE. (Kastenbaum, Robert, ed. Aging and Old Age Series.) Arno, New York. 1979.

30. Knopf, Olga. SUCCESSFUL AGING. G. K. Hall, Boston, Mass. 1977.

Sympathetically written by a physician who herself is facing the challenges of aging, this book contains gentle advice on retirement, use of leisure time, volunteer work, sexual adaptation, keeping fit, and dealing with aged parents. The early and later signs of aging are discussed, as are some of the qualities shared

by aged persons such as their deep need for independence, their fear of death, and their fear of pain.

31. Kurtzman, Joel, and Gordon, Philip. NO MORE DYING:
THE CONQUEST OF AGING AND EXTENSION OF HUMAN LIFE.
Dell, New York. 1977.

Shades of Ponce de Leon! This book acquaints the
reader with the more esoteric techniques gaining attention in man's relentless pursuit of youth. The
author investigates high technology, transplants, bi-
onics, cryobiology, and genetic engineering. It offers
an interesting discussion of doctors who specialize in
"youth" techniques.

32. Lamb, Lawrence E. STAY YOUTHFUL AND FIT: A DOCTOR'S
GUIDE. Harper & Row, New York. 1974.

33. Levinson, Daniel; Darrow, Charlotte N.; Kline, Edward
B.; Levinson, Maria H.; and McKee, Braxton. THE
SEASONS OF A MAN'S LIFE. Ballantine, New York. 1979.

The authors ask some crucial questions. What does it
mean to be an adult? What are the root issues of adult
life, the essential problems and satisfactions, the
sources of disappointment, grief, and fulfillment? Is
there an underlying order in the progression of our
lives over the adult years, as there is in childhood and
adolescence? Grappling with questions of this kind, the
authors ten years ago undertook a program of research,
and this book reports the progress they have made in
answering them.

34. McKenzie, Sheila C. SIXTY-FIVE AND BEYOND: AGING AND
OLD AGE. Scott, Foresman, Glenview, Ill. 1980.

35. Martin, Jane L., and DeGrucy, Clare. SWEEPING THE
COBWEBS. (Kastenbaum, Robert, ed. Aging and Old Age
Series.) Arno, New York. 1979.

36. Minot, Charles S. THE PROBLEM OF AGE, GROWTH, AND
DEATH. (Kastenbaum, Robert, ed. Aging and Old Age
Series.) Arno, New York. 1979.

37. Moss, Gordon, and Moss, Walter. GROWING OLD. Pocket
    Books, New York. 1975.

38. Saul, Shura. AGING: AN ALBUM OF PEOPLE GROWING OLD.
    Wiley, New York. 1974.

39. Schuckman, Terry. AGING IS NOT FOR SISSIES.
    Westminister Press, Philadelphia. 1975.

    This affirmative book simply states the author's prac-
    tical program for dealing with aging in a positive way.

40. Shanks, Ann Z. OLD IS WHAT YOU GET: DIALOGUES ON AGING
    BY THE OLD AND THE YOUNG. Viking, New York. 1976.

    In this beautifully illustrated text, the author inter-
    views a typical cross-section of American people and
    reveals the fears and attitudes of the old on matters
    of death, life, relationships, and remarriage. Comments
    from sensitive teenagers add another dimension.

41. Smith, Elliott D. HANDBOOK OF AGING. Barnes & Noble,
    New York. 1973.

    This book is directed to a number of people: the aged,
    those about to embark on old age, and professionals,
    relatives, or friends concerned with the care of the
    elderly. The author presents an unemotionally honest
    understanding of aging and reminds readers of important
    points to consider when reflecting on aging.

42. Stiegliz, Edward J. THE SECOND FORTY YEARS.
    (Kastenbaum, Robert, ed. Aging and Old Age Series.)
    Arno, New York. 1979.

43. Taylor, Florence M. YOU DON'T HAVE TO BE OLD WHEN YOU
    GROW OLD. Logos International, Plainfield, N.J. 1979.

44. Tibbitts, Clark. LIVING THROUGH THE OLDER YEARS.
    (Kastenbaum, Robert, ed. Aging and Old Age Series.)
    Arno, New York. 1979.

45. Turk, Ruth. YOU'RE GETTING OLDER, SO WHAT? Herald
Publishing House, Independence, Mo. 1976.

The author dispels many of the myths surrounding old
age and deals essentially with the feelings and problems
of the middle class. Very supportive for those spry
seniors.

46. Watson, Wilbur. STRESS AND OLD AGE. Transaction Books,
New Brunswick, N.J. 1979.

47. Abbo, Fred E. STEPS TO A LONGER LIFE. World Publications, Mountain View, Calif. 1979.

This book by a primary care specialist condenses a
large number of complex theories on preventive medicine
into an easy-to-follow guide. The author's prime
motivation in writing this book was to eliminate unnecessary and recurring doubts, fears, and questions
of his patients.

48. Aero, Rita. THE COMPLETE BOOK OF LONGEVITY. Putnam,
New York. 1979.

49. Bender, Ruth. BE YOUNG AND FLEXIBLE AFTER THIRTY, FORTY,
FIFTY, SIXTY ... Ruben Publishing, Avon, Conn. 1976.

50. Benet, Sula. HOW TO LIVE TO BE ONE HUNDRED: THE LIFE
STYLE OF THE PEOPLE OF THE CAUCASUS. Dial, New York.
1976.

This fascinating and historical account of an area in
southeastern Russia, where centenarians are as common
as joggers are here, is written by an experienced
anthropologist. The author studies the Caucasus region
from Greek and Roman times and examines its geographic,
ecologic, family, and community structures. Benet
shares with his readers an enlightening interview with
a spry, alert, 140 year old woman.

51. Cantor, Alfred U. DOCTOR CANTOR'S LONGEVITY DIET: HOW
TO SLOW DOWN AGING AND PROLONG YOUTH AND VIGOR.
Prentice-Hall, Englewood Cliffs, N.J. 1967.

This book offers lengthy consultations designed to re-
vitalize the body by a nutritionist and distinguished
surgeon of 40 years. The reader learns to strengthen
and restore energy where necessary, restore youth where
possible, prolong life in many cases, and enjoy a
healthier, more vital lifestyle. The author's practical and holistic approach is presented in a detailed
and easy to follow program.

52. Carlin, Joseph M. FOOD SERVICE GUIDE TO THE NUTRITION
PROGRAM FOR THE ELDERLY. New England Gerontology
Center, Durham, N.H. 1975.

53. Cornero, Luigi. THE ART OF LIVING LONG. (Kastenbaum,
Robert, ed. Aging and Old Age Series.) Arno, New
York. 1979.

54. Duke, Cecil Edward. HOW TO BE YOUNG AT SIXTY: THE
FOUNTAIN OF YOUTH. Exposition Press, Hicksville,
N.Y. 1975.

55. Flatto, Edwin. LOOK YOUNG, THINK CLEARER, LIVE LONGER.
Plymouth Press, Miami Beach, Fla. 1978.

56. Frank, Benjamin S., and Miele, Philip. DR. FRANK'S
NO-AGING DIET: EAT AND GROW YOUNGER. Dial, New York.
1976.

The author clearly explains to the reader the premise
for his extensive research in the dietary importance of
nucleic acids. With simple recipes this book shows how
nucleic acid-rich diets can aid drug addicts, alcoholics,
and those suffering from heart disease and osteo-
arthritis.

57. Fredericks, Carlton. LOOK YOUNGER, FEEL HEALTHIER.
(Orig. title: Eating Right for You.) Grosset & Dunlap,
New York. 1975.

Touching on a wide variety of topics relating to eating
habits and good nutrition, Fredericks discusses food
additives, vitamins, and nutrition in prevention and
treatment of diseases such as diabetes and mental illness. The book includes practical information on diet
plans, how to lose weight, how to make nutritious bread,
and how to shop in a health-food store.

58. Galton, Lawrence. HOW LONG WILL I LIVE? Pinnacle
Books, Los Angeles. 1977.

59. Gomez, Joan. HOW NOT TO DIE YOUNG. Stein & Day,
    Briarcliff Manor, N.Y. 1972.

    This book discusses potential health problems which
    can arise from the impairment of heart and arteries,
    lung and breathing apparatus, kidneys and bladder, and
    other physiological functions.

60. Gore, Irene. ADD YEARS TO YOUR LIFE AND LIFE TO YOUR
    YEARS. Stein & Day, Briarcliff Manor, N.Y. 1975.

    Vitality, not youth, is the keyword in this book. The
    author attempts to present in some detail the underlying
    ideas and evidence for her positive attitude toward ag-
    ing. The book offers practical suggestions for ways to
    achieve better health and greater vitality.

61. Hauser, Gayelord. LOOK YOUNGER, LIVE LONGER. Fawcett,
    New York. 1977.

62. Hill, Grace. FITNESS FIRST: PHYSICAL EXERCISES FOR ALL
    AGES. Hill, Hanover, N.H. 1979.

63. Hill, Howard E. NINE MAGIC SECRETS OF LONG LIFE.
    Prentice-Hall, Englewood Cliffs, N.J. 1979.

64. Homola, S. DOCTOR HOMOLA'S LIFE EXTENDER HEALTH GUIDE
    SECRETS THAT HELP YOU LIVE LONGER. Prentice-Hall,
    Englewood Cliffs, N.J. 1975.

65. Hrachovec, Josef P. KEEPING YOUNG AND LIVING LONGER.
    Sherbourne, Nashville, Tenn. 1972.

66. Hurdle, J. Frank. DOCTOR HURDLE'S PROGRAM TO RETAIN
    YOUTHFULNESS. Prentice-Hall, Englewood Cliffs, N.J.
    1972.

    This book asks the question: How would you like to look,
    feel, and stay younger? The author attempts to show how
    to do so with surprisingly little effort and without
    gimmicks or magic elixirs. The importance of body
    metabolism, physical conditioning, creative thinking,
    inner circles, and many other topics are discussed.

67. Kavanagh, Terence. HEART ATTACK? COUNTERATTACK!
    Van Nostrand Reinhold, New York. 1976.

68. Keyes, Kenneth S. LOVING YOUR BODY. (HOW TO LIVE
    LONGER, STRONGER, SLIMMER.) Frederick Fell Publishers,
    New York. 1974.

69. Kordel, Lelord. STAY ALIVE LONGER. 2nd ed. Manor
    Books, New York. 1977.

    The author, known for his natural folk remedies, pro-
    poses methods to revitalize health and preserve it with
    exercise and nutrition.

70. Kordel, Lelord. YOU'RE YOUNGER THAN YOU THINK. Popular
    Library, New York. 1979.

71. Kugler, Hans J. DR. KUGLER'S SEVEN KEYS TO A LONGER
    LIFE. Fawcett, New York. 1979.

    What is the ideal diet for longevity and for prevention
    of senility, heart attacks, and cancer? Dr. Kugler
    offers his concepts and advice and includes a longevity
    quiz to estimate one's personal life expectancy.

72. Leonard, Jon N., and Taylor, Elaine A. LIVE LONGER NOW
    COOKBOOK FOR JOYFUL HEALTH AND LONG LIFE. Grosset &
    Dunlap, New York. 1977.

    This cookbook is intended to teach the art of longevity
    through wise eating. The authors pinpoint the enemies
    in our diet as fats, sugars, salt, caffeine, and choles-
    terol. To avoid these, special help is offered in plan-
    ning vegetarian meals. Also included are numerous
    tables, glossaries, and menus.

73. Lewis, Clara M. NUTRITIONAL CONSIDERATIONS FOR THE
    ELDERLY. Davis Publication, New York. 1978.

74. Lumiere, Cornel. FEELING YOUNGER LONGER. Lyle Stuart,
    Secaucus, N.J. 1973.

75. Maness, William. EXERCISE YOUR HEART. Macmillan, New
    York. 1969.

76. Miller, Jonas E. PRESCRIPTION FOR TOTAL HEALTH AND
    LONGEVITY. Logos International, Plainfield, N.J. 1979.

77. McKenna, Marylou. REVITALIZE YOURSELF: THE TECHNIQUES
    OF STAYING YOUTHFUL. Hawthorn Books, New York. 1972.

    In this comprehensive and medically researched volume
    on body and mental conditioning, the author advises the
    reader on such topics as diets, hair health, stress,
    and sex.

78. McQueen-William, Morvyth, and Appisson, Barbara. A DIET
    FOR ONE HUNDRED HEALTHY, HAPPY YEARS. Prentice-Hall,
    Englewood Cliffs, N.J. 1977.

    Dr. McQueen-William's personal thirty-year battle with
    cancer and his extensive work in southeastern USSR, an
    area known for large numbers of centenarians, have en-
    abled this distinguished academic to co-author a fascin-
    ating informative book on longevity. Some excellent
    Armenian recipes are supplied.

79. Peters, Helen Hall. PHYSICAL FITNESS AND MENTAL HEALTH
    BEFORE AND AFTER RETIREMENT. Exposition Press,
    Hicksville, N.Y. 1977.

80. Posner, Barbara M. NUTRITION AND THE ELDERLY.
    Lexington Books, Lexington, Mass. 1979.

81. Rhodes, Russell L. MAN AT HIS BEST--HOW TO BE MORE
    YOUTHFUL, VIRILE, HEALTHY, AND HANDSOME. Doubleday,
    New York. 1974.

82. Richardson, Joseph G. LONG LIFE AND HOW TO REACH IT.
    (1st published Lindsay & Blakiston, Phila. 1879.)
    Edited by Barbara G. Rosenkrantz. Arno, New York. 1977.

    Written at the turn of the century, this amazingly
    timely book discusses such topics as sunstroke, clothing,
    and health.

83. Root, Leon, and Kiernan, Thomas. THE BAD BACK EXERCISE
    BOOK. Warner Books, New York. 1979.

84. Rosenberg, Magda. SIXTY-PLUS AND FIT AGAIN EXERCISES
    FOR OLDER MEN AND WOMEN. G. K. Hall, Boston, 1978.

85. Rothenberg, Robert. HEALTH IN THE LATER YEARS. New
    American Library, New York. 1972.

86. Sage, J. A. LIVE TO BE ONE HUNDRED AND ENJOY IT.
    Cornerstone Library, New York. 1975.

87. Shell, Adeline G., and Reynolds, Kay. FEEL BETTER AFTER
    FIFTY FOOD BOOK. Sovereign Books, New York. 1978.

    This book originated from an experimental workshop for
    older people in Queens, New York, called the Feel-Better
    Group. Its sole purpose was to help older people feel
    better by eating better. The authors feel this simple,
    straightforward approach to eating abets longevity.

88. Stonecypher, D. D., Jr. GETTING OLDER AND STAYING YOUNG.
    Norton, New York. 1974.

89. Taylor, Renee. HUNZA HEALTH SECRETS FOR LONG LIFE AND
    HAPPINESS. Keats Publishing, New Canaan, Conn. 1978.

90. Ticktin, George B. HOW TO BE ONE HUNDRED YEARS YOUNG.
    Frederick Fell, New York. 1979.

    Based on a series of lectures on longevity, the author
    contends that health maintenance is the key to long life
    and discusses the influence of sex, sleep, lifestyle,
    and other factors on longevity.

91. Weiner, Albert. DOCTOR WEINER'S MIRACLE DIET FOR HEALTH
    AND LONGEVITY. Prentice-Hall, Englewood Cliffs, N.J.
    1978.

92. Winick, Myron, ed. NUTRITION AND AGING. Wiley, New
    York. 1976.

    This book takes the position that nutrition during the
    early and middle years of life may be a crucial factor
    in determining both the rate of aging and the actual
    physiologic make-up of old age. The book attempts to
    examine the value of nutrition during early life and
    its effects on aging and, conversely, how the process
    of aging affects nutritional requirements.

The Science of Aging

93. Adams, George. ESSENTIALS OF GERIATRIC MEDICINE.
Oxford University Press, New York. 1978.

The author relates the value of science of general
medicine with the art of geriatrics in this tightly
written volume. The book highlights and discusses in
technical but comprehensible language important considerations in geriatric, medical, and clinical practice.

94. Anderson, W. Ferguson. PRACTICAL MANAGEMENT OF THE
ELDERLY. 3rd ed. Lippincott, New York. 1976.

This book is a practical guide to help physicians interested in the care of elderly patients.

95. Atchley, Robert C. SOCIAL FORCES IN LATER LIFE: AN
INTRODUCTION TO SOCIAL GERONTOLOGY. 2nd ed. Wadsworth,
Belmont, Calif. 1977.

This brief but comprehensive introduction to the subject
of human aging emphasizes its social and sociopsycho-
logical aspects. The book examines the multidisciplinary field dealing with social gerontology and summarizes
current knowledge about the impact of aging on biological and psychological functioning. The author deals with
situations that usually face aging individuals and discusses how society treats its older members.

96. Brown, Warren J. A DOCTOR'S ADVICE TO FOLKS OVER FIFTY.
Aero-Medical Consultants, Largo, Fla. 1976.

97. Carlisle, Anthony. AN ESSAY ON THE DISORDERS OF OLD AGE
AND ON THE MEANS FOR PROLONGING HUMAN LIFE. (Kastenbaum,
Robert, ed. Aging and Old Age Series.) Arno, New York.
1979.

98. Falconer, Mary W.; Altamura, Michael V.; and Behnke,
Helen Duncan. AGING PATIENTS: A GUIDE FOR THEIR CARE.
Springer, New York. 1976.

This book is designed as a quick reference for those persons involved in the care of the aging--professional
nurses, licensed practitioners, nurses' aides, social

workers, physical and occupational therapists. The book
emphasizes common physical and mental disorders of older
people and makes observations to correct or arrest the
progress of degenerative diseases. The author discusses
actions which professionals and communities can take to
help older citizens regain and keep their health.

99. Hahn, H. P. PRACTICAL GERIATRICS. S. Karger, White
Plains, N.Y. 1975.

100. Hall, Granville S. SENESCENCE, THE LAST HALF OF LIFE.
Arno, New York. 1972.

101. Hess, Patricia, and Day, Sandra. UNDERSTANDING THE
AGING PATIENT. R. J. Brady, Bowie, Md. 1977.

This book approaches geriatric nursing holistically
presuming that social and psychic facts are intimately
linked to physical disorders. This multidimensional approach is based on an understanding of the interaction
of multiple systems. The authors give special attention
to nursing care, communication, and mental disorders
along with a discussion of common diseases of old age.

102. Hodkinson, H. M. AN OUTLINE OF GERIATRICS. Academic,
New York. 1974.

103. Lewis, Sandra C. THE MATURE YEARS: A GERIATRIC
OCCUPATIONAL THERAPY TEXT. Charles B. Slack, Thorofare,
N.J. 1979.

104. Reichel, William. CLINICAL ASPECTS OF AGING. Williams
& Wilkins, Baltimore, Md. 1978.

The author writes for the practicing physician and other
allied health professionals who care for the elderly.
This practical volume focuses on the geriatric patient
and emphasizes pitfalls to be avoided in the daily care
of the elderly.

105. Rossman, Isadore, ed. CLINICAL GERIATRICS. 2nd ed.
Lippincott, New York. 1979.

106. Schwartz, Arthur N., and Peterson, James A. INTRODUCTION
TO GERONTOLOGY. Holt, Rinehart & Winston, New York. 1979

107. Worcester, Alfred. THE CARE OF THE AGED, THE DYING
     AND THE DEAD. 2nd ed. (1st published 1950.) Arno,
     New York. 1976.

     This book presents a very sensitive, humanistic ap-
     proach to the care of the aged, the dying, and the dead.
     It can serve as an excellent supplement to the physi-
     cian's library.

Mental Health and Aging

108. Bellak, Leopold, and Karasu, T., eds. GERIATRIC
PSYCHIATRY: A HANDBOOK FOR PSYCHIATRISTS AND PRIMARY
CARE PHYSICIANS. Grune & Stratton, New York. 1976.

109. Burnside, Irene M. PSYCHOSOCIAL NURSING CARE OF THE
AGED. McGraw-Hill, New York. 1972.

A comprehensive treatment of nursing and aging, this
book includes discussions of the normal aging process
and deviations of pathophysiology in the elderly which
have implications for nursing care. Research on aging
is described.

110. Butler, Robert N., and Lewis, Myrna I. AGING AND MENTAL
HEALTH: POSITIVE PSYCHOSOCIAL APPROACHES. 2nd ed.
Mosby, St. Louis, Mo. 1977.

The aim of this highly sensitive book is to provide
students of gerontology, as well as the general reader,
with an understanding of old age and a sense of the
historical growth in the field. The authors write in
a style that is comprehensible and free of jargon while,
at the same time, introducing the basic terminology of
the field. The book discusses the nature and problems
of old age and deals with prevention, treatment, and
evaluation. The appendices include valuable sources of
gerontological and geriatric literature, organizations
pertaining to the elderly, governmental programs for the
elderly, grant programs, and social services.

111. Fann, William E., and Maddox, George. DRUG ISSUES IN
GEROPSYCHIATRY. Williams & Wilkins, Baltimore, Md.
1974.

112. Frankfather, Dwight. THE AGED IN THE COMMUNITY:
MANAGING SENILITY AND DEVIANCE. Praeger, New York.
1977.

The author probes the social realities of everyday life
for the senile person. By analyzing 14 treatment settings from mental hospitals and nursing homes to the
fire department and corner cafeteria in one middle-sized
eastern community, Dr. Frankfather discovers that the

professional community is out of touch with the very
people it is striving to help.

113. Garfield, Charles A., ed. STRESS AND SURVIVAL: THE
     EMOTIONAL REALITIES OF LIFE THREATENING ILLNESS. Mosby,
     St. Louis, Mo. 1979.

114. Gershon, S., and Raskin, A., eds. GENESIS AND TREATMENT
     OF PSYCHOLOGIC DISORDERS IN THE ELDERLY. Raven, New
     York. 1975.

     Hoping to create a new cross-discipline--geriatric
     psychobiology--the authors have gathered contributions
     on research in the treatment of psychologic disorders
     in the elderly. This valuable reference book is in-
     tended for students, clinicians, and specialists.

115. Lawton, George, ed. NEW GOALS FOR OLD AGE. Arno,
     New York. 1972.

     The editor hopes this contribution will change the
     community's prevailing attitude about older people
     which, in turn, will lead to the expansion and improve-
     ment of facilities for the aged. This book is a collec-
     tion of papers which shares some recent ideas concerning
     the nature and needs of older people.

116. Lowenthal, Marjorie F., and Berkman, Paul L. AGING AND
     MENTAL DISORDER IN SAN FRANCISCO: A SOCIAL PSYCHIATRIC
     STUDY. Jossey-Bass, San Francisco. 1967.

117. Pitt, Brice M. PSYCHOGERIATRICS: AN INTRODUCTION TO
     THE PSYCHIATRY OF OLD AGE. Churchill Livingstone,
     New York. 1974.

118. Savage, R. D.; Britton, P. G.; Bolton, N.; and Hall,
     E. H. INTELLECTUAL FUNCTIONING IN THE AGED. Methuen,
     New York. 1973.

     The investigations discussed in this book were under-
     taken with the cooperation of the elderly people of
     Newcastle upon Tyne, from 1963 to 1971. Several major
     problems addressed are the assessment of and develop-
     mental changes in intellectual functioning in the
     community's aged and in the mentally ill aged; and

the problems of intellectual impairment in the elderly
in relation to clinical diagnosis and survival.

119. Simon, Alexander; Lowenthal, Marjorie Fiske; and Epstein,
     Leon J. CRISIS AND INTERVENTION: THE FATE OF THE ELDERLY
     MENTAL PATIENT. Jossey-Bass, San Francisco, 1970.

     This book describes a universe of older urban residents
     who were hospitalized with serious psychiatric disturb-
     ances during one calendar year. The sociological, psy-
     chological, psychiatric, and physical health factors
     involved in the admission of older people to psychi-
     atric facilities are studied and the spectrum of normal
     and abnormal aging processes analyzed from an inter-
     disciplinary point of view.

120. Verwoerdt, Adrian. CLINICAL GEROPSYCHIATRY. Williams
     & Wilkins, Baltimore. 1976.

121. Whitehead, J. A. PSYCHIATRIC DISORDERS IN OLD AGE:
     A HANDBOOK FOR THE CLINICAL TEAM. Springer Publishing,
     New York. 1974.

     The team approach to treatment and support in psychiatry
     and geriatrics is highly fashionable and may in time
     extend to other branches of medicine. Whitehead's
     volume is a practical handbook for geriatricians,
     family doctors, students, and all members of any team
     that should be involved in providing services for old
     people with psychiatric illness. The text, enlivened
     by case histories, demonstrates the beneficial effects
     of active team therapy, and provides details of other
     services currently available to the psychogeriatric
     patient.

ALCOHOLISM AND DRUG ABUSE

From the beginnings of recorded history, human beings have used substances to help them transcend the bounds of reality. Alcohol and other mind-altering drugs have been the chemical agents that have provided for this transcendence. Society's reaction to problems arising from unhealthy practices with drug use has been more a function of legality than a product of pharmacology.

Alcohol, with the exception of the 14 years of Prohibition, has been the accepted legal drug of choice for social use. Other chemical agents are controlled or restricted by a variety of legal and medical restraints.

The history of alcohol and other drug use is replete with expressions of moral outrage by a population that considered the use of external aids to alter consciousness evidence of characterological weakness. Problems resulting from the overuse and dependence on these substances have kindled the momentum for social outrage. The majority of people, however, use these products beneficially and safely; but a relatively few (7 percent of the population) become controlled by and addicted to these substances.

Success with the technology to control infectious diseases by isolating and eliminating the causative agents served to offer policymakers a simple answer to a complex problem. The U.S. Congress, reacting to this theory, voted the only amendment to the constitution ever repealed, the 18th amendment mandated the elimination of alcohol. This experiment in control and restriction not only proved to be a catastrophic failure but facilitated the advent of organized crime.

Cross-cultural studies of societies with a similar physical, social, economic, and emotional makeup show no appreciable problems among the population with either alcohol or drugs. Today, with new knowledge and findings, treatment programs and prevention efforts have forged in new directions toward reducing substance abuse.

Government supported research and treatment efforts have shown that treatment for alcoholism and drug abuse is effective. However, health professionals tend to avoid making a diagnosis that labels people alcoholics or addicts and often set up measures for treatment success that guarantee failure. People with alcohol or other drug problems, when provided with customized care, recover at rates equal to recovery rates from other treatable illnesses.

Researchers and policy developers have begun to ask the larger question: What is there about life today that requires the increasing use of mind-altering drugs? The use of substances is "learned behavior" usually imparted by family role models. Although some substance abuse experts feel that an abnormal dependence on substances may be caused by a physical or genetic defect, most likely a complicated, complex intertwining of a variety of factors sows the seeds of alcoholism and drug abuse.

As new information and research pour into these areas, exciting opportunities for innovative treatment and prevention efforts become possible.

ALCOHOLISM AND DRUG ABUSE

General

122. Amit, Zalman, and Sutherland, E. Ann. GUIDE TO
INTELLIGENT DRINKING. Walker & Co., New York. 1977.

This book has a specific audience in mind: problem
drinkers--not alcoholics nor social drinkers--but people
who have become concerned about the amount of alcohol
they consume.

123. Anderson, Daniel J. THE JOYS AND SORROWS OF SOBRIETY.
Hazelden, Center City, Minn. 1977.

124. Beck, Sandy. THE ALCOHOLIC'S GUIDE TO SOBRIETY AND
RECOVERY. Ermine Publications, Hollywood, Calif. 1977.

This book is a response to the author's own needs to
evolve a positive philosophy and approach which facilitated his successful recovery from alcoholism. This
guide is recommended for anyone who needs help with an
alcohol problem. The author points out how physicians,
law enforcement officers, and attorneys can successfully
get to the heart of the alcohol problem of many people
with whom they deal professionally.

125. Becker, Charles E.; Roe, Robert L.; and Scott, Robert A.
ALCOHOL AS A DRUG. Krieger Publications, Huntington,
N.Y. 1979.

This volume is a comprehensive treatise on the pharmacology, neurology, and toxicology of alcohol as a drug.
It was prepared by a group of physicians who have considerable scientific expertise and a humanistic concern
about the effects of alcohol. The authors write about
the biobehavioral aspects of alcohol abuse and its
treatment and critically examine a number of intervention techniques. This critical and thoughtful review
of the literature coupled with the authors' own experience is a refreshing approach.

126. Bennett, A. E. ALCOHOLISM AND THE BRAIN. Stratton, New York. 1977.

127. Block, Marvin A. ALCOHOL AND ALCOHOLISM: DRINKING AND DEPENDENCE. Wadsworth, Belmont, Calif. 1970.

128. Blum, K., ed. ALCOHOL AND OPIATES: NEUROCHEMICAL AND BEHAVIORAL MECHANISMS. Academic Press, New York. 1977.

This comprehensive overview addresses the commonalities and distinctions of alcohol and opiate use and misuse within a framework that emphasizes both neurochemical and behavioral mechanisms.

129. Carroll, Charles R. ALCOHOL: USE, NONUSE, AND ABUSE. Wm. C. Brown, Dubuque, Iowa. 1975.

130. Chafetz, Morris E., and Demone, Harold W., Jr. ALCOHOLISM AND SOCIETY. Oxford University Press, New York. 1962.

This volume examines the causes of alcoholism and reviews previous works on the subject, including defini-
tions of alcoholism, psychological theories, and other
related scientific research. The role of drinking is
related to attitudes toward alcoholism in different
cultures. The book views the work conducted by such
programs as Alcoholics Anonymous and the Yale Center of
Alcohol Studies, and examines concepts and methods of
alcoholism prevention. The appendices include a bibliography and eleven case histories.

131. Cormier, Edmond. HOPE, HOPELESSNESS AND THE ALCOHOLIC. Hazelden, Center City, Minn. 1978.

132. Edwards, Griffith, and Grant, Marcus, eds. ALCOHOLISM. NEW KNOWLEDGE AND NEW RESPONSES. (Revised papers of a meeting held in Sept. 1976, at the Institute of Psychiatry, London.) University Park Press, Baltimore. 1977.

133. Filstead, William, J.; Rossi, J. J.; and Keller, M.,
     eds. ALCOHOL AND ALCOHOL PROBLEMS: NEW THINKING AND
     NEW DIRECTIONS. Ballinger, Cambridge, Mass. 1976.

     This monograph examines the current state of knowledge
     in the alcohol field, finds it lacking, and offers pro-
     vocative and challenging suggestions for change. The
     authors critically analyze the inability of the field
     to meet the challenges of alcohol problems.

134. Fort, Joel. ALCOHOL: OUR BIGGEST DRUG PROBLEM.
     McGraw-Hill, New York. 1973.

     This book ascribes antisocial conduct to the beer, wine,
     and spirits industry and indicts them as pushers of al-
     cohol. The author cautions the reader to use alcohol
     as discriminatingly as possible while discussing alter-
     nate sources of pleasure and meaning.

     A public health specialist and criminologist, the author
     has crusaded nationally and internationally to have al-
     cohol recognized as the greatest public health issue in
     the nation. He advises a public health brand of treat-
     ment and prevention rather than rejection and criminal-
     ization for alcoholics and other drug abusers.

135. Freed, Earl X. AN ALCOHOLIC PERSONALITY? C. B. Slack,
     Thorofare, N.J. 1979.

136. Galanter, Marc, ed. CURRENTS IN ALCOHOLISM. Vol. VI.
     Academic Press, New York. 1979.

     Papers delivered to an annual conference on alcoholism
     constitute this volume. In the section on treatment,
     general hospital, in-patients, and medically ill alco-
     holics are discussed. In the section on rehabilitation,
     papers describe follow-up studies on patients who have
     had psychotherapy or who have been members of Alcoholics
     Anonymous. Adolescents, women, and drunken drivers are
     discussed in the epidemiology section.

137. Glatt, Max. ALCOHOLIC AND THE HELP HE NEEDS. Taplinger,
     New York. 1974.

     The author's presentation of personal experiences with
     British alcoholics observed during two decades in a

variety of settings affords the reader a realistic appraisal and understanding of the difficulties confronting the alcoholic.

The book stresses the value of special units in hospitals for the treatment of alcoholics as outpatients and addresses the need to treat each sufferer with patience, sympathy, understanding, and firmness. The author strongly urges the structure of a good aftercare program.

138. Gust, Dodie. FACE TO FACE WITH ALCOHOLISM. Hazelden, Center City, Minn. 1979.

The author gives a complete and lucid explanation of confrontation therapy and explains how it works in alcoholism. This new technique, which offers hope for recovery, has some suggestions of harshness. The author's presentation is nonjudgmental.

139. Haberman, Paul W., and Baden, Michael. ALCOHOL, OTHER DRUGS AND VIOLENT DEATH. Oxford University Press, New York. 1978.

140. Hafen, Brent Q. ALCOHOL: THE CRUTCH THAT CRIPPLES. West Publishing, St. Paul, Minn. 1977.

This book helps the reader understand: 1) the use of alcoholic beverages in American society; 2) the physical and social effects of alcoholic beverages; 3) problem drinking and alcoholism; and 4) prevention and treatment of alcohol problems. The book draws heavily on research reports published by the National Institute of Mental Health (NIMH) and the National Institute on Alcohol Abuse and Alcoholism (NIAAA) and may be used as a text for courses in the social and health sciences.

141. Harper, Frederick D., ed. ALCOHOL ABUSE AND BLACK AMERICA. Douglass, Alexandria, Va. 1976.

142. Johnson, Vernon. I'LL QUIT TOMORROW: A BREAKTHROUGH TREATMENT FOR ALCOHOLISM. Harper & Row, New York. 1973.

143. Judge, Bill C. THE AGONY OF ALCOHOLISM AND HOW I
     OVERCAME IT. Exposition Press, Hicksville, N.Y. 1979.

144. Keller, John E. DRINKING PROBLEM. Fortress,
     Philadelphia. 1971.

145. Kessel, Neil, and Walton, Henry. ALCOHOLISM. Penguin,
     New York. 1966.

     This book about alcoholism, written by two experienced
     psychiatrists, focuses on the harmful aspects of alcohol
     misuse. The authors are well versed in scientific re-
     search and have the gift of translating complex findings
     and jargon into lucid and interesting prose. The phys-
     ical, psychological, and social aspects of alcoholism
     are all considered and some principles of treatment and
     prevention are explained.

146. Klewin, Jane, and Klewin, Thomas. WHEN THE MAN YOU LOVE
     IS AN ALCOHOLIC. Abbey Press, St. Meinrad, Indiana.
     1979.

147. Linn, Robert. YOU CAN DRINK AND STAY HEALTHY. Watts,
     New York. 1979.

     Dr. Linn, an authority on nutritional medicine, has
     written a guide for the social drinker. He offers a
     complete program of diet, nutrition, and exercise that
     allows one to drink and stay healthy. A number of fac-
     tors which are the bases for the guide are discussed,
     for example, how alcohol affects the body, especially
     the brain, and how drinking affects weight, sex life,
     appearance, and the way one ages. He offers advice on
     how to cope with the morning-after and discusses the
     question of whether or not drinking can help prevent
     heart attacks.

148. Lord, Eileen, and Lord, Luther. HOW TO COMMUNICATE IN
     SOBRIETY. Hazelden, Center City, Minn. 1976.

     This book explores the self-destructive personality
     characteristics of passivity and hostility as they
     relate to recovery from alcoholism. Through clever
     illustrations and sound sensible directives, the
     authors, who have worked many years with recovering

alcoholics, teach the problem drinker strategies to enable them to take charge of their lives.

149. Maloney, Ralph. TWENTY-FOUR HOUR DRINK BOOK. Astor-
Honor, New York. 1962.

150. McCabe, Thomas. VICTIMS NO MORE. Hazelden, Center
City, Minn. 1978.

This book addresses an often-forgotten fact: problem
drinkers are not the only victims of alcoholism;
spouses, children, and others suffer devastating pain
and emotional loss. Dr. McCabe offers hope for freedom
and a new way of life to these often-neglected individuals. This volume explains how family members may un-
consciously perpetuate the drinking, and it provides a
step-by-step method of confronting the drinker with an
awareness of his destructive behavior. The author contends that an examination of rational-emotive techniques
will show how changing the way one thinks about drinking
can change the way one feels about it.

151. Mann, Marty. MARTY MANN ANSWERS YOUR QUESTIONS ABOUT
DRINKING AND ALCOHOLISM. Holt, Rinehart & Winston,
New York. 1970.

152. Mariken, Gene, and Scheinmann, Eugene. A DOCTOR'S
SENSIBLE APPROACH TO ALCOHOL AND ALCOHOLISM. Budlong
Press, Chicago. 1969.

153. Mehl, Duane. YOU AND THE ALCOHOLIC IN YOUR HOME.
Augsburg, Minneapolis. 1979.

The author, a recovered alcoholic, knows how to deal
with the problems of alcoholism realistically and effectively. He writes about money, sex, counseling,
social drinking, and prescription drugs; and describes
in nontechnical language the drugs popular among
today's youth. He explores treatment programs for alcoholics as well as companion groups for members of an
alcoholic's family.

154. Meyer, Lewis. OFF THE SAUCE. Macmillan, New York.
     1976.

     This book relates the story of one man's life on and off
     "the sauce." The author's only mission is to comfort
     alcoholics and non-drinkers, preferably recovered drink-
     ers and members of Alcoholics Anonymous.

155. Milt, Harry. ALCOHOLISM: ITS CAUSES AND CURE. Scribner,
     New York. 1976.

156. Nathan, Peter E.; Marlatt, G. Alan; and Koberg, Tor,
     eds. ALCOHOLISM: NEW DIRECTIONS IN BEHAVIORAL RESEARCH
     AND TREATMENT. Ser. III. Human Factors, Vol. 7.
     Plenum, New York. 1978.

157. Paolino, Thomas J., and McCrady, Barbara S. THE
     ALCOHOLIC MARRIAGE: ALTERNATIVE PERSPECTIVES. Grune,
     New York. 1977.

     The single most influential and motivating force in
     writing this book was the authors' concern that many
     mental health clinicians and researchers manifest pro-
     found sophistication in one perspective or school of
     thought but, simultaneously, show only superficial
     familiarity with viewpoints alien from their own. Dif-
     ferent theoretical scientific perspectives of alcoholic
     marriages are offered.

158. Patten, G. Z. YOU, TOO, CAN STOP DRINKING. Exposition
     Press, Hicksville, N.Y. 1977.

     The 20 chapters in this book are the 20 lectures which
     resulted from the author's work at Mountaintop Center
     in Tennessee, a rehabilitation facility for male prob-
     lem drinkers. Lectures written in a sensitive manner
     are based on the 12 steps taken by Alcoholics Anonymous.

159. Reilly, Richard L.   AMERICA'S WORST DRUG PROBLEM:
     ALCOHOL. Liguori Publications, Liguori, Mo. 1974.

160. Reilly, Richard L.   I'M NOT AN ALCOHOLIC BECAUSE.
     Liguori Publications, Liguori, Mo. 1979.

161. Royce, James E. ALCOHOL AND RESPONSIBILITY. Hazelden,
     Center City, Minn. 1979.

162. Shipp, Tom. THE TROUBLE WITH ALCOHOL. Revell, Old
     Tappan, N.J. 1978.

     This book tries to serve as a bridge across the present
     gap between lay groups like Alcoholics Anonymous and
     professionals in the field of alcoholism. The author
     attempts to guide alcoholics, who are forced to choose
     between experts or lay persons, to find the help they
     need from both groups. The author makes a plea to other
     ministers and professionals who work with alcoholics not
     to take alcohol away from troubled people until they
     give them something to replace it, i.e., self respect
     and the assurance of God's love, and faith in their fel-
     low human beings.

163. Shore, Richard, and Luce, John M. TO YOUR HEALTH: THE
     PLEASURES, PROBLEMS AND POLITICS OF ALCOHOL. Seabury
     Press, New York. 1976.

     The major difference between pleasure drinkers and
     problem drinkers is that the former wish to expand
     awareness and the latter wish to confine it. The
     authors' primary purpose in writing the book is to in-
     crease society's awareness of and respect for this much-
     maligned subject, alcohol.

164. Sobell, Linda C., ed. EVALUATING ALCOHOL AND DRUG ABUSE
     TREATMENT EFFECTIVENESS. Pergamon, Elmsford, N.Y.
     1979.

     This book presents a coherent set of analyses regarding
     problems of alcohol and drug addictions associated with
     treatment, treatment evaluation and methodologies em-
     ployed. Useful suggestions are offered for improving
     the quality of evaluation studies.

165. Steiner, Claude. GAMES ALCOHOLICS PLAY. Ballantine,
     New York. 1977.

     Steiner, a disciple of the late Eric Berne, offers hope
     for the problem drinker. By analyzing life scripts and
     using an extension of the theory and practice of

transactional analysis, he believes he can offer a more
effective treatment for alcoholism and other addictions.
The alcoholic, he maintains, is driven by an inner com-
pulsion for self-destruction. Through case histories
of alcoholics and their treatment, he unfolds his ideas.

166. Steiner, Claude. HEALING ALCOHOLISM. Grove, New York.
1979.

This book is written for alcoholics, their families, and
their friends. Steiner maintains that alcoholism is not
a disease but a bad habit. The roles of nutrition and
bodywork are emphasized in his suggested treatment.

167. Strack, Jay. DRUGS AND DRINKING: THE ALL AMERICAN
COP-OUT. Nelson, Nashville, Tenn. 1979.

The concern for America's youth, so clearly evident in
this book, comes both from the author's beginnings in a
family shattered by alcohol and from his own years of
drug abuse. The book strips away the mystery of drug
and alcohol abuse among the young and offers easy-to-
understand accurate information and insights necessary
to help penetrate the confusion of today's youth. Excellent resource for counselors, pastors, educators,
and parents.

168. Tracy, Don. WHAT YOU SHOULD KNOW ABOUT ALCOHOLISM.
Dodd, Mead, New York. 1975.

This book is the result of the New Life Foundation's
concern about the dearth of practical information on
ways nonalcoholics can recognize and help loved ones,
friends, and employees stricken with alcoholism. This
book is an assemblage of responses to a questionnaire
sent to the families and friends of alcoholics.

169. Weiner, Jack. DRINKING. Norton, New York. 1976.

170. Weston, Drake. GUIDEBOOK FOR ALCOHOLICS: HOW TO
SUCCEED WITHOUT DRINKING. Exposition Press,
Hicksville, N.Y. 1964.

171. Wilkerson, Don. FAST TRACK TO NOWHERE. Revell, Old
     Tappan, N.J. 1979.

     The author has witnessed the devastating effects that
     alcohol has on its victims, especially among teenagers
     for whom alcohol has become the drug of choice. Based
     on his counseling experience of more than 18 years, the
     author has written this book to help parents and teach-
     ers alike in solving this serious problem.

172. Wilkinson, Rupert. PREVENTION OF DRINKING PROBLEMS:
     ALCOHOL CONTROL AND CULTURAL INFLUENCES. Oxford Univ.
     Press, New York. 1970.

173. Williams, Robert J. ALCOHOLISM: THE NUTRITIONAL
     APPROACH. University of Texas Press, Austin, Texas.
     1959.

174. Willoughby, Allan. THE ALCOHOL TROUBLED PERSON.
     Nelson-Hall, Chicago. 1979.

Alcoholism in the Workplace

175. Beyer, Janice M., and Trice, Harrison M. IMPLEMENTING
CHANGE: ALCOHOLISM IN WORK ORGANIZATIONS. Free Press,
New York. 1978.

This book reports on a study of a legislative effort
designed to implement change on the issue of alcoholism
in the workplace. The research focuses on deliberate
and planned change rather than spontaneous change. The
authors discuss the change process, sampling, data collection, statistics, stages of implementation, roles of
directions, and interorganizational relations.

176. Brisolara, Ashton. THE ALCOHOLIC EMPLOYEE: A HANDBOOK
OF HELPFUL GUIDELINES. Human Science Press, New York.
1978.

177. Follmann, Joseph F., Jr. ALCOHOLICS AND BUSINESS:
PROBLEMS, COSTS, SOLUTIONS. New ed. American Management, New York. 1976.

The purpose of this book is to view the effects of alcoholism and problem drinking on the business community,
on industrial management, on employees, and organized
labor, as well as on health and welfare funds and on
insurance programs.

178. Plant, Martin A. DRINKING CAREERS: OCCUPATIONS,
DRINKING HABITS AND DRINKING PROBLEMS. Methuen, New
York. 1979.

179. Schramm, Carl J., ed. ALCOHOLISM AND ITS TREATMENT IN
INDUSTRY. Johns Hopkins, Baltimore, Md. 1977.

The papers assembled here have been selected by the
editor, whose experience in developing teaching materials for the course "The Problems of Work" at the Johns
Hopkins School of Hygiene and Public Health brought him
into close contact with the contributors of the book.
His role in directing a multi-employee, multi-union
clinic in Baltimore for employed alcoholics has made
him an expert on employee alcohol programs.

180. Schramm, Carl J.; Mandell, Wallace; and Archer, Janet.
     WORKERS WHO DRINK. Lexington Books, Lexington, Mass.
     1978.

181. Trice, Harrison M., and Roman, Paul M. SPIRIT AND
     DEMONS AT WORK: ALCOHOL AND OTHER DRUGS ON THE JOB.
     2nd ed. New York School of Industrial Relations,
     Cornell University, Ithaca, N.Y. 1979.

     This book deals with the job behaviors of alcoholics and
     other drug abusers. The authors use the constructive
     confrontation strategy as a tool for motivating people
     into help. A major contribution of this book is the ex-
     cellent analysis and redesign of programs offering al-
     ternatives and new approaches for female employees.

182. Wrich, James T. THE EMPLOYEE ASSISTANCE PROGRAM.
     Hazelden, Center City, Minn. 1974.

183. Burtle, Vasanti. WOMEN WHO DRINK: ALCOHOLIC EXPERIENCE
AND PSYCHOTHERAPY. C. C Thomas, Springfield, Ill.
1979.

184. Coney, John C. EXPLORING THE KNOWN AND UNKNOWN FACTORS
IN THE RATES OF ALCOHOLISM AMONG BLACK AND WHITE
FEMALES. R&E Research Assn., Palo Alto, Calif. 1978.

Despite the fact that the problem of alcoholism is gaining notice both nationally and internationally, little
attention has been given to alcohol abuse among black
females. Much confusion exists in the literature re-
garding alcohol abuse among the total black population.
There appears, however, to be a consensus of an increase in alcoholism among black females. This book
discusses many of the problems, methodologies, and current literature in this area.

185. Curlee-Salisbury, Joan. WHEN THE WOMAN YOU LOVE IS AN
ALCOHOLIC. Abbey Press, St. Meinrad, Indiana. 1979.

This book is written for a vast audience of husbands,
brothers, sisters, sons, daughters, grandchildren, and
friends who live with an alcoholic and are bewildered
by the seemingly contradictory dictates of love in a
highly confusing situation.

186. Fajardo, Rogue. HELPING YOUR ALCOHOLIC BEFORE HE OR SHE
HITS BOTTOM. Crown, New York. 1976.

This book explodes the myth that an alcoholic cannot be
helped unless he or she wants help. It spells out positive actions the spouse of an alcoholic can take to cope
with problems and thereby bring about basic changes in
an alcoholic marriage.

187. Hornik, Edith L. THE DRINKING WOMAN. Follett, New
York. 1978.

Women have been neglected subjects in alcoholism research but recent studies are finding physiological
differences in their reactions to alcohol. The rhythm
of their lives, goals, and their interaction with

society, spouses, and children are all different from those of men. This book will be welcome encouragement for those who seek treatment and who need the knowledge to obtain it.

188. Leite, Evelyn. TO BE SOMEBODY. Hazelden, Center City, Minn. 1979.

The author shows the truth of the Al-Anon observation that those who love and live with a drinking alcoholic become victims of the illness also. The book weaves a story about alcoholism and pain, about faith in a higher power and healing of the soul, about joy and recovery--from an Al-Anon point of view.

189. Sandmaier, Marion. THE INVISIBLE ALCOHOLIC. McGraw-Hill, New York. 1980.

The text focuses exclusively for the first time on the growing problem of alcohol abuse by women. Stigmatizing attitudes toward the drinking woman affect her dealings with men, marriage, sex, her children, and her job. The author reveals why women drink and why treatments designed for men don't work for women--and what does work. Included are a Woman's Guide for obtaining assistance for a drinking problem, a list of helping organizations, and national information sources.

190. Wortitz, Janet G. MARRIAGE ON THE ROCKS: HOW TO LIVE WITH AN ALCOHOLIC. Delacorte, New York. 1979

191. Youcha, Geraldine. A DANGEROUS PLEASURE. Hawthorn, New York. 1978.

The author attempts to provide information rather than polemics about a subject that triggers deeply personal responses. The book explores research, opinion, and human experience to present an up-to-date picture of what is known about the effects of drinking on women.

Alcohol Problems and Drug Abuse
Among Teenagers and Children

192. Alibrandi, Tom. YOUNG ALCOHOLICS. CompCare Publications, Minneapolis. 1978.

This book offers a practical plan of action--not just reaction--for any adult trying to cope with a problem-drinking child or adolescent. The author, director of youth programs for the Council on Alcoholism, Orange County, California, suggests ways to determine when a youngster is in trouble--or about to be in trouble--with alcohol.

193. Blane, Howard T., and Chafetz, Morris E., eds. YOUTH, ALCOHOL AND SOCIAL POLICY. Plenum, New York. 1979.

The contributors to this edited book provide an updated statement on the epidemiology of drinking behavior incorporating data which correlates drinking with sex, age and other demographic characteristics. Social policy implications of youthful drinking practices are examined in detail and, finally, programs designed to promote the responsible development of pragmatic and beneficial social action are reviewed.

194. Cross, Wilbur. KIDS AND BOOZE: WHAT YOU MUST KNOW TO HELP THEM. Dutton, New York. 1979.

This book is for the reader whose son or daughter has a drinking problem. It helps the reader focus on the nature of the problem and determine steps to take to correct it. The author does not expound on medical, psychological, or social theories nor expose the reader to scare stories or horror tales. He just writes a down-to-earth book on a serious subject.

195. Englehardt, Stanley L. KIDS AND ALCOHOL, THE DEADLIEST DRUG. Lothrop, Lee & Shepard, New York. 1975.

196. Fleming, Alice. ALCOHOL: THE DELIGHTFUL POISON. Dell, New York. 1979.

197. Haskins, Jim. TEEN-AGE ALCOHOLISM. Hawthorn, New York.
     1976.

     Using the attractive method of true and false questions,
     Haskins explains the facts and corrects misconceptions
     about alcohol and the drinking habit. Questions dis-
     cussed include whether beer is less intoxicating than
     whiskey, whether taking cold showers and drinking strong
     coffee after drinking help to sober one up, and whether
     drinking helps or hinders sexual performance.

198. Hornik, Edith L. YOU AND YOUR ALCOHOLIC PARENT.
     Association Press, New York. 1973.

     This book explores parental behavior and alcoholism.
     Descriptions of the way alcoholism manifests itself in
     family life are given, followed by explanations of these
     manifestations which become understandable even when
     they are not forgivable. The book ends with a descrip-
     tion of Alateen--the special organization for teenagers
     with alcoholic parents--and many other community re-
     sources available for help, understanding, and friend-
     ship.

199. Langone, John. BOMBED, BUZZED, SMASHED, OR ... SOBER.
     Avon, New York. 1979.

     This practical, provocative book is informative and
     educational. Hundreds of questions about drinking are
     answered, such as: Is coffee the best way to sober up?
     Does liquor in any quantity have a bad effect on the
     body? Is alcoholism an illness? How many drinks make
     a person drunk? What is the right way to drink? Is
     there a difference between a problem drinker and an
     alcoholic? Also included is a glossary of alcoholic
     beverages.

200. Lyles, John S. YOUTH AND ALCOHOLIC BEVERAGES. John
     Knox, Atlanta. 1967.

201. Marshall, Shelly, ed. YOUNG, SOBER AND FREE. Hazelden,
     Center City, Minn. 1978.

     This practical book sets forth in disarming and some-
     times irreverent fashion the harsh truth about young

people and mind-affecting chemicals. The authors relate the personal experiences of those who have lived
through addiction. The work also furnishes a clear
picture of the primary tools of recovery--the twelve
steps of Alcoholics Anonymous.

202. Mayer, John, and Filstead, William, eds. ADOLESCENCE
AND ALCOHOL. Ballinger, Cambridge, Mass. 1979.

203. Milgram, Gail G. ALCOHOL EDUCATION MATERIALS: AN
ANNOTATED BIBLIOGRAPHY. Rutgers Center for Alcohol
Studies, New Brunswick, N.J. 1975.

204. North, Robert J., and Orange, Richard A., Jr. TEENAGE
DRINKING: THE NUMBER ONE DRUG PROBLEM IN AMERICA TODAY.
Macmillan, New York. 1980.

This book was written primarily as a potential tool for
teenagers to learn more about teenage drinking. The
authors have attempted to integrate information with
ideas, to separate myth from fact, and to combine humor
with the seriousness the subject requires. It is especially useful for parents, teachers and youth workers,
and contains useful appendices that offer additional
suggestions for initial intervention.

205. Seixas, Judith S. LIVING WITH A PARENT WHO DRINKS TOO
MUCH. Greenwillow, New York. 1979.

This book was written to help children of alcoholics
understand what is happening to them and their parents.

206. Snyder, Anne. MY NAME IS DAVY. I'M AN ALCOHOLIC.
Holt, Rinehart and Winston, New York. 1977.

This book describes the sensitive, painful story of a
teenager's victorious battle over alcohol.

207. Wagnen, Robert. SARAH T.: PORTRAIT OF A TEENAGE
ALCOHOLIC. Ballantine, New York. 1976.

FITNESS AND EXERCISE

The everyday demands of a rural society have automatically managed the fitness needs of its population, but
with the advent of urbanization and technology, the automatic balance between intake and output deteriorated. The
need of people to actively seek exercise for the well-being
of their bodies precipitated the birth of a new cottage
industry: the pursuit of fitness.

The body contains some 650 muscles that operate on a
fundamental principle: use them or lose them. Unused
healthy muscles begin to lose strength and substance; and
within a short time, they become weak, sluggish, and
withered. Moreover, since human beings rose up on their
hind legs some million years ago to take the first tenta-
tive step, the need to walk has become a crucial element
to well-being.

Hippocrates, the father of medicine, considered walking
a person's best medicine. Exercise by walking or by other
physical action is vital to the maintenance of a fit body
and mind. Hippocrates was the first to emphasize how intimately the mind and body functioned as a unit. An un-
fortunate by-product of the celebration of freedom from
drudgery provided by technology and affluence is indolence.
Indolence has led to overindulgence, overindulgence to
sluggish bodies and minds.

The precipitous rise in the incidence of lifestyle-
related diseases has alarmed and sobered concerned individuals; consequently, the nation has seen an unprecedented
surge of interest in the pursuit of physical fitness.
Joggers, runners, walkers, sports enthusiasts, and health
club habitues attest to the growing awareness that people
are ready and willing to accept some responsibility for
their health and well-being.

A regular regime of exercise stimulates the circula-
tion, increases the body's temperature, aids in the effective operation of a strong and healthy heart, aids the
efficient distribution of oxygen, and increases the capacity of the lungs. Exercise increases fitness, balances

appetite, and weight, and provides the physical capacity
to do more for longer periods.

Although the physical benefits of exercise are substantial, the mental rewards are equally impressive. The
daily business of living exposes people to an everpresent
threat to well-being: stress. The results of stress
contribute to a considerable number of illnesses. Many
techniques to attenuate the harmful effects of stress
have been developed, but none surpasses the stress-reduction
benefits of vigorous exercise.

FITNESS AND EXERCISE

Fitness and Choices

208. Agress, Clarence M. ENERGETICS. Grosset & Dunlap, New York. 1978.

The author explains the science of energetics and teaches the reader of any age how to harness inner vital force through exercise. Chapters include tennis and other racket sports, exercise and the heart patient, and Dr. Agress' thirteen-day diet.

209. Allen, Evlyn. FIGURING IT OUT: DIET AND EXERCISE FOR A LOVELIER YOU. Horizon, Bountiful, Utah. 1977.

The information on weight reduction in this book can be applied to any diet prescribed by a doctor. It stresses complete physical and emotional rehabilitation and long-range aspects of problems before and after weight loss. The author includes some interesting recipes.

210. Allen, Jean, and Mix, Emily S. BUILD A BETTER--AND SLIMMER--YOU. Arlington House, New Rochelle, N.Y. 1977.

211. Anderson, Bob. STRETCHING. Anderson Kramer, Washington, D.C. 1975.

212. Annarino, Anthony A. DEVELOPMENTAL CONDITIONING FOR WOMEN AND MEN. 2nd ed. C. V. Mosby, St. Louis. 1976.

This book, based on valid research evidence, describes and illustrates a variety of conditioning programs. Introductory material provides the physical education teacher, athletic coach, trainer, physical therapist, and athlete with a set of scientific foundations and principles for guidance in designing a specific conditioning program.

213. Astrand, P. O. HEALTH AND FITNESS. Barron, Woodbury, N.Y. 1977.

The author, the noted Swedish authority on physical fitness and aerobic exercise, explains clearly and enthusiastically how our bodies respond to exercise.

214. Bailey, Covert. FIT OR FAT. Houghton-Mifflin, Boston. 1978.

215. Barr, Beverly. I'D LIKE TO SEE LESS OF YOU. Atheneum, New York. 1975.

216. Beinhorn, George, ed. FOOD FOR FITNESS. World Publications, Mountain View, Calif. 1975.

217. Boff, Vic. YOU CAN BE PHYSICALLY PERFECT, POWERFULLY STRONG. Arco, New York. 1975.

The author appeals primarily to the male reader and offers information on a wide range of topics which includes sleep, diet, conditioning, muscle-building programs, and posture.

218. Bolton, Elizabeth, and Goodwin, Diane. POOL EXERCISES. 4th ed. Churchill Livingston, Edinburgh, Scotland. 1974.

This book attempts to scientifically explain the importance of pool therapy in the treatment of locomotor disability. The authors present a plan for a series of progressive exercises that should prove valuable to anyone interested in the techniques of pool therapy.

219. Briggs, George M., and Calloway, Doris H. BOGERT'S NUTRITION AND PHYSICAL FITNESS. 10th ed. Saunders, Philadelphia. 1979.

This well-researched and documented book, useful for the university-level nutrition student, presents the basic facts and principles of nutrition in a simple and interesting manner.

220. Cooper, Kenneth. AEROBICS. Bantam, New York. 1972.

221. Cooper, Kenneth. THE AEROBICS WAY. Bantam, New York. 1978.

Dr. Cooper originally began writing to counteract the problems of American lethargy and inactivity. From a more motivational approach, he is now concentrating on offering guidelines for exercise specially age-adjusted to the capabilities of men, women, and children. Suitable exercises are detailed for the pregnant woman, the cardiac patient, and the over-forty individual. Safeguards and tips are provided to manage and overcome minor but troublesome problems which might otherwise deter one from following or continuing the exercise program.

222. Cooper, Mildred, and Cooper, Kenneth. AEROBICS FOR WOMEN. Bantam, New York. 1973.

223. Covino, Marge, and Jordan, Pat. WOMEN'S GUIDE TO SHAPING YOUR BODY WITH WEIGHTS. Lippincott, New York. 1978.

In this "body-building" book, the authors hope to dispel forever the macho myth that lifting weights is not a feminine activity. This well-illustrated book describes preparatory exercises and explains techniques and equipment needed to begin this fitness program.

224. Craig, Marjorie. MISS CRAIG'S FACE-SAVING EXERCISES. Random House, New York. 1970.

In this "face-saving" program, the author designs exercises that offset the aging effects of gravity and counterbalance "set expression" patterns which weaken facial muscles. Excellent drawings of all facial muscles accompany the exercises.

225. Craig, Marjorie. MISS CRAIG'S TWENTY-ONE DAY SHAPE UP PROGRAM FOR MEN AND WOMEN. Random House, New York. 1968.

Exercises for everyone in search of a trim and healthy body are effectively illustrated with clear photographs in this book. Exercises for post-pregnancy are also presented. A system of check-off boxes provides a record of day-to-day performance.

226. Craig, Marjorie. MISS CRAIG'S 10-MINUTE A DAY SPOT
     REDUCING PROGRAM. Random House, New York. 1979.

     This beautifully illustrated book has the same woman
     model for the photographs of exercises as portrayed in
     the author's previous successful books on exercise. A
     catalogue of exercises for improving specific parts of
     the body is given, ranging from the fingers to the
     total body. Also taken into account is the fact that
     people often have limited space for performing these
     exercises.

227. Crawford, Benny. BOOK FOR EVERY BODY. World
     Publications, Mountain View, Calif. 1979.

     This concise encyclopedia is an exercise book to shape,
     tone, strengthen, and tighten every muscle in the body.
     In addition to exercises especially designed for men
     and women, the author, a champion body builder and a
     former Mr. California, offers exercises for couples,
     children, off-season athletes, and expectant mothers.

228. D'Asero, Barbara. BE YOUNG AND VITAL: THE NUTRITION
     EXERCISE PLAN. Enslow Publ., Short Hills, N.J. 1979.

229. Diagram Group. THE COMPLETE ENCYCLOPEDIA OF EXERCISES.
     Paddington, New York. 1979.

     This unique and complete volume offers tests to assess
     and rate fitness, explains reasons for the different
     forms of exercise, and details the benefits derived
     from each of them. Exercises range from those for
     general health, weight reduction, and pregnancy through
     body building and sports, to yoga and jogging, as well
     as techniques for mental relaxation to relieve tension
     and stress. Official national programs of the U. S.
     President's Council on Physical Fitness, the Health
     Education Council of Great Britain, and the People's
     Republic of China are included.

230. Doan, Daniel. DAN DOAN'S FITNESS PROGRAM FOR HIKERS AND
     CROSS-COUNTRY SKIERS. New Hampshire Publishing,
     Sommersworth, N.H. 1978.

     New Hampshire's eminent outdoorsman, Daniel Doan,

explains his special program for a healthful, active
outdoor life. Clear instructions and true-to-life
drawings show people of all ages and all levels of
physical fitness reasonable step-by-step isometric,
calisthenic, and endurance exercises to keep in shape.

231. Feldenkrais, Moshe. AWARENESS THROUGH MOVEMENT: HEALTH
     EXERCISES FOR PERSONAL GROWTH. Harper & Row, New York.
     1977.

     The author deals with the total person—physically,
     mentally, and psychologically—and concentrates on the
     individual's often hazy or distorted self-image.
     Grouped into 12 lessons, exercises consist of simple,
     easy, slow movements designed to reduce force and in-
     crease sensitivity.

232. Filson, Sidney, and Jessup, Claudia. JUMP INTO SHAPE:
     THE FAST, FUN WAY TO PHYSICAL FITNESS. Watts, New York.
     1978.

233. Flatto, Edwin. LOOK YOUNGER, THINK CLEARER AND LIVE
     LONGER. Plymouth Press, New York. 1978.

234. Garrison, Linda; Leslie, Phyllis; and Blackmore,
     Deborah. FITNESS AND FIGURE CONTROL: THE CREATION OF
     YOU. Mayfield Publ., Palo Alto, Calif. 1974.

235. Gault, Jim. THE WORLD OF WOMEN'S GYMNASTICS. Celestial
     Arts, Millbrae, Calif. 1976.

     Jim Gault has written a stimulating, sensitive and
     sometimes provocative book on artistic gymnastics. The
     author guides a youngster from the first day in a gym-
     nasium to participation on an International Gymnastics
     Team at the World Games. The book will be of interest
     to gymnasts, coaches, judges, parents of gymnasts,
     teachers, and the enthusiastic gymnastic spectator.

236. Gillie, Oliver, and Mercer, Derrik, eds. THE SUNDAY
     TIMES BOOK OF BODY MAINTENANCE. The Sunday Times
     Magazine, London. 1978.

     This delightful book on body maintenance is a British
     import. Packed with supurb illustrations and photos,

this entirely new kind of guide to health from childhood to old age offers a lifestyle to all members of the
family to improve their health, and outlines ways to
identify problems before they become serious. Done
with the inimitable grace, style, and wit indigenous to
the English, the Sunday Times presents a remarkably
entertaining and informative book.

237. Hegne, Barbara. EVERYWOMAN'S EVERY DAY EXERCISE AND
NUTRITION BOOK. Keats, New Canaan, Conn. 1979.

238. Hill, Grace. FITNESS FIRST: PHYSICAL EXERCISES FOR ALL
AGES. Grace Hill, Hanover, N.H. 1979

239. Hinrichsen, Gerda. THE BODY SHOP: SCANDINAVIAN EXER-
CISES FOR RELAXATION. Barnes & Noble, New York. 1977.

The author discusses simple methods for correcting
posture while working, walking, standing, and sitting.
This clearly written text, which includes well-illustrated exercises in conscious relaxation, analyzes tension
and the benefits of relaxation.

240. Horkey, Robert V. PHYSICAL FITNESS: THE PATHWAY TO
HEALTHFUL LIVING. 3rd ed. Mosby, St. Louis, Mo. 1977.

The author helps the readers evaluate their present
level of physical fitness and presents the necessary information to support the importance of physical activity.

241. Johnson, Barry L., and Garcia, Mary J. CONDITIONING:
FITNESS AND PERFORMANCE FOR EVERYONE. Rev. ed.
Sterling Swift, Manchaca, Texas. 1978.

242. Johnson, Bruce L. CHINESE WAND EXERCISE. Morrow, New
York. 1979.

Borrowing some secrets of the ancients, this book describes the use of the Chinese wand. Well-illustrated
with photographs, the book includes both standing and
floor exercises and offers a program to reduce fat, tone
muscles, stimulate the cardiovascular system, and improve
one's poise, posture, and agility. The author claims
that the exercises are safe for all ages.

243. Kahn, Manya. MANYA KAHN'S BODY RHYTHMS: FOR A
     HEALTHIER...LOVELIER...MORE DESIRABLE YOU. Dutton,
     New York. 1977.

     This book is the expression of the author's philosophy
     derived from a life of working with thousands of women
     of all ages, first as a dancer and teacher of dance,
     then as a student of physical therapy, and now as a
     teacher of physical fitness. This book shows how body
     rhythms work in conjunction with proper breathing, re-
     laxation, and diet to develop potential for vitality
     and liveliness.

244. Kuntzleman, Charles. THE EXERCISER'S HANDBOOK. McKay,
     New York. 1978.

245. Kuntzleman, Charles T., and Consumer Guide Editors.
     RATING THE EXERCISES. Penguin, New York. 1980.

     This book rates the current crop of fitness programs and
     helps the reader determine how much exercise is needed.
     The ratings assigned in this book are based on the
     authors' conclusion that cardiovascular type exercise is
     best for heart, muscles, body weight, and appearance.

246. Lebo, Fern. THE EVERY OTHER DAY EXERCISE BOOK: THE
     EASY-DOES-IT PROGRAM FOR BETTER BODIES. Stein & Day,
     Briarcliff Manor, N.Y. 1977.

     This book provides complete, accurate and up-to-the-
     minute essentials required for maintaining physical fit-
     ness. The author, a physiotherapist, discusses low back
     pain, prenatal and postnatal exercises, and exercises
     for post heart attack.

247. Lepanto, James D., and Jenkins, F. Compton. EXERCISE:
     FOR THE HEALTH OF IT. Kendall-Hunt, Dubuque, Iowa.
     1978.

248. Lowen, Alexander, and Lowen, Leslie. THE WAY TO VIBRANT
     HEALTH. Harper & Row, New York. 1977.

     The authors claim that this manual of bioenergetic exer-
     cises is a way of understanding one's personality in
     terms of the body and its energetic processes. Both

body and mind must work together to help resolve emotional problems. Thus, this exercise program is offered
as a form of therapy. The exercises are clearly illustrated with line drawings.

249. Man, John. WALK! IT COULD CHANGE YOUR LIFE.
Paddington, New York. 1979.

250. Mann, George V., and Garret, H. Leon. OVER 30: AN
EXERCISE PROGRAM FOR ADULTS. Aurora, Nashville, Tenn.
1970.

In outlining and explaining his program for attaining
physical fitness, the author answers such questions as:
What is the best activity? What is safe? Where and at
what time of day should one exercise? What about obesity and diets? What about existing ailments, medications, and medical precautions? How does one measure
progress?

251. Marten, Michael, and Chesterman, John. MAN TO MAN: NEW
ANSWERS TO OLD QUESTIONS ABOUT YOUR HEALTH, FITNESS AND
SEXUALITY. Paddington, New York. 1978.

252. Michener, Leslie, and Donaldson, Gerald. THE EXERCISE
BOOK. Holt, Rinehart & Winston, New York. 1978.

Ms. Michener, a physical education professional, demonstrates her complete program of exercises using color
and black and white photographs. Each of the 48 movement patterns involves a sequence of positions that
incorporates some combination of strengthening, stretching and/or relaxing different groups of muscles.

253. Minick, Michael. KUNG FU: HEALTH SECRETS OF ANCIENT
CHINA. Simon & Schuster, New York. 1974.

254. Mitchell, Curtis. THE PERFECT EXERCISE: THE HOP, SKIP
AND JUMP WAY TO HEALTH. Pocket Bks., New York. 1978.

255. Morehouse, Lawrence E., and Gross, Leonard. TOTAL
FITNESS IN THIRTY MINUTES A WEEK. Simon & Schuster,
New York. 1976.

Over a million copies of this book are already in print.

Morehouse claims that fitness is a "piece of cake," and offers ways to lose weight forever in a program of short steps that involve only thirty minutes a week. Fifteen fitness myths are described and dispelled.

256. Paul, Mark. THE TV EXERCISE BOOK. Dale Books, Waterbury, Conn. 1979.

257. Percival, Jan; Percival, Lloyd; and Taylor, Joe. THE COMPLETE GUIDE TO TOTAL FITNESS. Methuen, New York. 1977.

This well-illustrated text explains basic fitness priorities and describes exercises to keep the body young. Lloyd Percival, a world-renowned fitness expert and coach, provides tests to determine personalized programs to meet individual strengths and weaknesses, offers a bank of exercises to draw on, methods for tackling particular physical faults, good eating habits, and ways to deal with tension at work and home.

258. Peters, Helen Hall. PHYSICAL FITNESS AND MENTAL HEALTH BEFORE AND AFTER RETIREMENT. Exposition Press, Hicksville, N.Y. 1977.

259. Prudden, Suzy, and Sussman, Jeffrey. FIT FOR LIFE. Macmillan, New York. 1978.

It is important to know that from the age of 24 onward your body produces fewer and fewer cells; youthfulness diminishes but it can be replaced with attractive vigor, health, and strength. The authors show you how to deal with your entire body, how to get back into shape, and how to stay there, while controlling particular problems. With minimal time, you should have a lean body, a strong heart, and the necessary endurance for a successful career, marriage, and life of leisure.

260. Root, Leon, and Kiernan, Thomas. THE BAD BACK EXERCISE BOOK. Warner Bks., New York. 1979.

The author of this book is a practicing orthopedic surgeon with years of experience in dealing with back problems. For this book, he has created 10 different specially formulated and illustrated exercise programs

for bad back victims in lieu of surgery or other forms
of medical therapy.

261. THE ROYAL CANADIAN AIR FORCE EXERCISE PLANS FOR PHYSICAL
     FITNESS. Pocket Bks., New York. 1976.

     This is a revised edition of the classic official Royal
     Canadian Air Force Exercise Program and is designed for
     both men and women. Hints on weight control, diet, and
     exercises for the heart are included along with a pro-
     gressive exercise program which is clearly illustrated
     with black silhouettes.

262. Schwarzenegger, Arnold. ARNOLD'S BODYSHAPING FOR WOMEN.
     Simon & Schuster, New York. 1979.

     Everything a woman could possibly want in the way of
     achieving a lifetime of fitness and beauty is promised
     in this progressive exercise program. How to reshape
     and change your body, firm up your thighs, reduce but-
     tocks, increase the bustline, flatten the stomach, and
     improve your posture are some of the targets. The
     author promises that these exercises are the fastest,
     most efficient way to shape up, trim down, feel great,
     and look terrific.

263. Shierman, Gail, and Haycock, Christine. TOTAL WOMAN'S
     FITNESS GUIDE. World Publ., Mountain View, Calif. 1979.

     The authors have gathered an impressive amount of in-
     formation any woman would need to know to begin or main-
     tain a personal program of fitness. This authoritative
     handbook was written by women for women who want to look
     better, feel better, and have fun in the process.

264. Smith, Ann. STRETCH! Acropolis, Washington, D.C. 1979.

265. Smith, David. THE EAST-WEST EXERCISE BOOK. McGraw-Hill,
     New York. 1976.

     This collection of exercises is adapted from a wide
     variety of international disciplines, including bio-
     energetics, yoga, mime, and Tai Chi. Step-by-step
     instructions for a five-cycle set of exercises and

exercises for special problem areas are illustrated
with photographs.

266. Smith, R. Philip. THE LA COSTA DIET AND EXERCISE BOOK.
Grosset & Dunlap, New York. 1977.

267. Solomon, Neil, and Harrison, Evalee. DOCTOR SOLOMON'S
PROVEN MASTER PLAN FOR TOTAL BODY FITNESS AND
MAINTENANCE. Berkley Publications, New York. 1978.

This book concentrates on key areas of the body--chest,
abdomen, arms, back, buttocks, feet and ankles, hips,
legs, knees, waistline, and midriff. Special exercises
are offered for sufferers from back pains. Advice is
included concerning sexual fitness and an excercise-
awareness program.

268. Spackman, Robert R. EXERCISE IN THE OFFICE: EASY WAYS
TO BETTER HEALTH AND FIRMER FIGURES. Southern Illinois
Univ. Press, Carbondale, Ill. 1969.

269. Speads, Carola H. BREATHING: THE ABCs. Harper & Row,
New York. 1978.

Step-by-step, the author guides the reader through the
various ways of improving breathing. The gentle exercise "experiments" in this book are simple and easy to
do, can be done anywhere, and require no special equipment.

270. Treber, Grace. SANASESSION: FOUR-MINUTE EFFORTLESS
INCHES OFF AND SLIMMING PROGRAM FOR MEN AND WOMEN.
Source Publ., New York. 1969.

Sanasession is a 4-minute program of effortless exercise
poses for men and women utilizing scientific movement
and timing to achieve a fit and beautiful body without
hard exercising and soreness. Excellent illustrations
and explanation accompany the routines.

271. Treber, Grace. SIX MINUTE SANA FACIAL EXERCISES FOR
MEN. Source Publ., New York. 1971.

272. Tulloh, Bruce. NATURAL FITNESS. Simon & Schuster,
New York. 1977.

273. Uram, Paul. THE COMPLETE STRETCHING BOOK. World
     Publ., Mountain View, Calif. 1979.

274. Ureldinger, Ron, and Richards, Lomerett. ISOROBICS:
     A BETTER WAY TO FITNESS. Whitmore, Ardmore, Pa. 1979.

275. Wiederanders, Rex E., and Addeo, Edmond G. BIOTONICS.
     Warner Bks., New York. 1978.

     The authors discuss how the biotonic strength and
     stamina program works. The book includes information
     on a range of motion exercise, muscle mechanics, breath-
     ing, and psychology of exercise, among other topics.

276. Yoels, Jennifer. RE-SHAPE YOUR BODY, RE-VITALIZE YOUR
     LIFE. Prentice-Hall, Englewood Cliffs, N.J. 1972.

277. Zohman, Lenore; Kattus, Albert A., and Softness, Donald
     G. THE CARDIOLOGIST'S GUIDE TO PHYSICAL FITNESS AND
     HEALTH THROUGH EXERCISE. Simon & Schuster, New York.
     1979.

     Based on a scientific understanding of exercise, this
     book helps the reader decide whether present physical
     activity is enough or excessive. The authors help the
     individual devise a personal program and show how to
     evaluate exercise programs in health clubs and spas
     and those described in books and magazines.

Jogging and Walking

278. Ald, Roy. JOGGING, AEROBICS, AND DIET. New American Library, New York. 1973.

279. Batten, Jack. THE COMPLETE JOGGER. Harcourt, Brace, Jovanovich, New York. 1977.

The author anticipates and answers a variety of questions about jogging. More than a physical fitness plan, the book combines chapters on how jogging affects the body, disposition and sex life, and talks about famous joggers of the past. It includes information on trivia, sleep routines, and score charts to tabulate body performance.

280. Bowerman, William J., and Harris, W. E. JOGGING. Ace Books, New York. 1978.

Jogging is free, easy, relaxing, fun, can be done alone or in groups, and is good for your heart and lungs, say the authors. Richly illustrated with photographs of people of all ages and sizes who jog, the book includes special pointers for women as well as a discussion of feet and proper shoes. A progress chart is included to guide the reader in a jogging program.

281. Dare, Bernie. RUNNING AND YOUR BODY: APPLYING PHYSI-OLOGY TO TRACK TRAINING. Tafnews Press, Los Altos, Calif. 1979.

282. Davis, John T. WALKING! Bantam, New York. 1979.

283. D'Alton, Martina. THE RUNNER'S GUIDE TO THE U.S.A. Summit Books, New York. 1979.

284. Donaldson, Gerald. THE WALKING BOOK. Holt, Rinehart & Winston, New York. 1979.

In this book, Donaldson does for walking what James Fixx did for running. The author explains the physiology of walking, compares its benefits to other aerobic exercises, and tells the reader how to do it better. Complete with provocative and amusing anecdotes about Roosevelt, Plato, Thoreau, and others, this book is an

entertaining look at how, why, where, and when to walk
whatever the person's age or physical condition.

285. Fixx, James F. THE COMPLETE BOOK OF RUNNING. Random
     House, New York. 1977.

     Jogging, according to Fixx, makes you feel better, be-
     come slimmer, live longer, drink and smoke less, have a
     better sex life, increase your self-esteem, and attain
     a state of serenity. This encyclopedic work includes
     everything from how to decide whether or not you are cut
     out to be a runner, what gear and diet are best, how to
     prepare for a marathon, and suggests a program for an
     individual who has suffered a previous heart attack.

286. Gale, Bill. THE WONDERFUL WORLD OF WALKING. William
     Morrow & Co., Inc., New York. 1979.

     Created to inspire and help men, women, and children
     enjoy the art of walking, the author shows how to build
     a regular walking program that will heighten sensory
     awareness and even change the way a person looks, feels,
     and thinks. The book describes what happens to your
     psyche and your body when you walk and how walking be-
     comes a tranquilizer, anti-depressant or a stimulant.
     In addition, clothes and shoes are discussed as well as
     the food and vitamins you should consume. Walking tours
     of twelve great American cities are included for the
     reader's enjoyment.

287. Geline, Robert J. THE PRACTICAL RUNNER. Macmillan,
     New York. 1978.

     This useful handbook is directed to the beginning or
     continuing runner who understands that running regularly
     is beneficial. The author discusses equipment, working
     out (excellent yoga exercises), weather, nutrition, and
     prevention of injuries.

288. Gilmore, Haydn. JOG FOR YOUR LIFE. New ed. Zondervan,
     Grand Rapids, Mich. 1979.

289. Heidenreich, Steve, and Dorr, Dave. RUNNING BACK. Hawthorn, New York. 1979.

The author writes a sensitive story about the physical and psychological rehabilitation of a runner with a promising running career as he recovers from a near fatal car accident.

290. Heinonen, Janet. SPORTS ILLUSTRATED RUNNING FOR WOMEN. Lippincott, New York. 1979.

This comprehensive guide is filled with the kind of coaching tips, practical advice, medical facts, and competitive know-how to develop good running habits. The author gives special consideration to problems of young runners, senior runners, overweight runners, and to areas of pregnancy, birth control, and the menstrual cycle.

291. Henderson, Joe. JOG, RUN, RACE. World Publications, Mountain View, Calif. 1977.

292. Hochman, Sandra. JOGGING: A LOVE STORY. Putnam, New York. 1979.

293. Hoffman, Robert, and Cantley, Jed. RUNNING TOGETHER: THE FAMILY BOOK OF JOGGING. Leisure Press, West Point, N.Y. 1979.

294. Kuntzleman, Charles T., and the Editors of Consumer Guide. THE COMPLETE BOOK OF WALKING. Wm. Morrow & Co., New York. 1979.

Charles T. Kuntzleman, a recognized expert in the field of physical fitness, and the editors of Consumer Guide have developed what just may be the easiest system ever devised to get people in shape and keep them there.

295. Lance, Kathryn. RUNNING FOR HEALTH AND BEAUTY. Bobbs-Merrill, Indianapolis, Indiana. 1977.

This book presents a complete medically responsible program for every level of runner who wants to improve health and appearance. It shows how to enjoy running regardless of age, physical condition, and lifestyle.

296. Olney, Ross R. THE YOUNG RUNNER. Lothrop, New York.
     1978.

     This book presents basic information for beginning
     runners and briefly discusses marathons, organizations,
     and equipment sources.

297. Runner's World Editors. NEW EXERCISE FOR RUNNERS.
     World Publications, Mountain View, Calif. 1978.

298. Sheehan, George. RUNNING AND BEING. Simon & Schuster,
     New York. 1978.

     In his book, Dr. Sheehan gives the reader his recipe for
     a lifetime program of fitness and joy showing how the
     body determines an individual's mental and spiritual
     energies; and, by building a healthy body, how people can
     rebuild a new life. Fitness is necessary, says Sheehan,
     if people are to find themselves, know self-respect, and
     to meet life's challenges.

299. Spino, Michael. THE INNER SPACES OF RUNNING: BEYOND
     JOGGING. Celestial Arts, Millbrae, Calif. 1976.

     The author revitalizes the monotony of jogging by intro-
     ducing the reader to an imaginative variety of tempos,
     styles, and visualization techniques that can make
     running a carnival of delights. Spino suggests medita-
     tion, energy awareness, and methods of Olympic coaches
     that can benefit beginners and skilled runners alike.

300. Spino, Michael. RUNNING HOME. Celestial Arts, Millbrae,
     Calif. 1977.

     The author's pioneering approach to running--an integra-
     tion of mind/body experience--is the basis for a com-
     plete fitness program for the entire family. Specific
     techniques include auxiliary running forms and gaits,
     Feldenkrais exercises, yoga postures, visualization,
     energy awareness, and concentration.

301. Ullyot, Joan, M.D. WOMEN'S RUNNING. World Publica-
     tions, Mountain View, Calif. 1976.

     Dr. Joan Ullyot writes that the hardest step for a woman
     who wants to run is the first one out the door because
     she has to lay aside all her old ways of thinking. The
     book pays special attention to the mature woman who runs
     for fitness and long-distance competition. It includes
     tips on shoes, clothing, diet, safety precautions for
     runners, medical advice, and research findings.

Conditioning for Sports

302. Englebardt, Stanley L. HOW TO GET IN SHAPE FOR SPORTS. Lothrop, New York. 1976.

303. Jennison, Keith, and Pratt, William A. YEAR-AROUND CONDITIONING FOR PART-TIME GOLFERS. Atheneum, New York. 1979.

304. Jensen, Clayne, and Fisher, A. Garth. SCIENTIFIC BASIS OF ATHLETIC CONDITIONING. 2nd ed. Lea & Fabiger, Philadelphia. 1979.

The book on conditioning and performance should be especially useful to coaches and teachers and to upper division and graduate students majoring in physical education. The authors present a wealth of information on conditioning guidelines and physiological factors affecting performance.

305. Leonard, George. THE ULTIMATE ATHLETE. Viking Press, New York. 1974.

The author's contention that an athlete lives within each of us is not an abstract concept but a belief that athletic ability can change the way we feel and live. The search for an inner athlete can result by participating in sports and regular exercise.

However, Leonard's thesis goes beyond health and fitness to a transcendence of the human body toward spiritual satisfaction. The book includes an examination of the mythology, history, and evolution of games and sports.

306. Levy, Allan M., and Welb, Allan. CONDITIONING FOR THE HIGH SCHOOL ATHLETE. Contemporary Books, Chicago. 1979.

This book gives a structured approach to conditioning for young athletes. The authors present sections on prevention of injury, mental attitudes, and use of weights. The three types of exercise dealt with are isometric, isokinetic, and isotonic.

307. O'Neill, Frank, and Libby, Bill. SPORTS CONDITIONING: GETTING IN SHAPE, PLAYING YOUR BEST AND PREVENTING INJURIES. Doubleday, New York. 1979.

308. Riordan, J. SPORT IN SOVIET SOCIETY. Cambridge Univ.
     Press, New Rochelle, N.Y. 1977.

309. Rosenthal, Gary. SPALDING GUIDE TO FITNESS FOR THE
     WEEKEND ATHLETE. Grosset & Dunlap, New York. 1978.

     This book presents a very easy and sensible way to get
     in shape and stay there.

310. Schurman, Dewey. ATHLETIC FITNESS; THE ATHLETE'S GUIDE
     TO TRAINING AND CONDITIONING. Atheneum, New York. 1975.

     The book outlines the training and conditioning methods
     practiced by today's top professional and amateur
     athletes. These techniques not only help improve
     athletic performance, but can make the difference be-
     tween a successful career in sports and a career cut
     short by injury.

311. Siegener, Ray. SHAPE UP FOR SPORTS. Berkley Publica-
     tions, New York. 1978.

312. Soderholm, Eric. CONDITIONING FOR BASEBALL. Anna
     Publications, Winter Park, Fla. 1978.

313. Spackman, Robert R., Jr. CONDITIONING FOR BASEBALL:
     PRE-SEASON, REGULAR SEASON AND OFF-SEASON. Charles C
     Thomas, Springfield, Ill. 1967.

314. Sprague, Ken. THE GOLD'S GYM BOOK OF STRENGTH TRAINING
     FOR THE DEDICATED ATHLETE. St. Martin's, New York.
     1979.

     This excellent manual for the serious athlete outlines
     individualized sports programs from aikido to kayaking
     to wrist wrestling.

315. Tokle, Art. THE COMPLETE GUIDE TO CROSS-COUNTRY SKIING
     AND TOURING. Random House, New York. 1977.

     This excellent updated classic discusses the techniques
     of cross-country skiing and the selection of equipment.
     It contains up-to-the-minute information on kinds of
     skis, bindings, boots, accessories, and their costs.

In addition, the author provides a complete listing of cross-country ski centers and accommodations across the country.

316. Todd, Terry, and Hoover, Dick. FITNESS FOR ATHLETES. Contemporary Books, Chicago. 1978.

317. Turner, Lowell, and Turner, Sue. CREATIVE EXPERIENCE THROUGH SPORTS. Peek Publications, Mountain View, Calif. 1978.

318. Unitas, John, and Dintiman, George B. IMPROVING HEALTH AND PERFORMANCE IN THE ATHLETE. Prentice-Hall, Englewood Cliffs, N.J. 1979.

This book fulfills a longstanding need in major sports, where misconception, myths, and dangerous practices plague an area that has become an important part of the American way of life. This text draws information from related areas in psychology, physiology, and sociology, practical knowledge, expert opinion, and research to provide answers to the questions and concerns of athletes, coaches, parents, and spectators.

319. Whitehead, N. CONDITIONING FOR SPORTS. Charles River Books, Boston. 1975.

This book provides a guide for coaches who plan schedules of conditioning or "fitness training" for the sportsmen and women in their care.

Fitness for Children

320. Barr, Beverly. EXERCISE GAMES FOR CHILDREN AND PARENTS. Sterling, New York. 1978.

321. Block, Susan D. ME AND I'M GREAT: PHYSICAL EDUCATION FOR CHILDREN THREE THROUGH EIGHT. Burgess, Minneapolis. 1977.

This guide for early childhood physical development out-lines a complete program of activities ranging from ap-paratus work to games and stunts. The book correlates the psychological and motor development of young chil-dren to the importance of physical education.

322. Bucher, Charles A., and Keonig, Constance R. METHODS AND MATERIALS FOR SECONDARY SCHOOL PHYSICAL EDUCATION. 5th ed. C. V. Mosby, St. Louis, Mo. 1978.

This revised text will enlighten and assist the college student in physical education, the physical educator, educators in general, and other persons interested in the field.

323. Coe, Boyer, and Sumner, Bob. GETTING STRONG, LOOKING STRONG: A GUIDE TO SUCCESSFUL BODYBUILDING. Atheneum, New York. 1979.

324. Corbin, Charles B. BECOMING PHYSICALLY EDUCATED IN THE ELEMENTARY SCHOOL. 2nd ed. Lea & Fabiger, Philadelphia. 1976.

The book is designed to aid the physical educator to ascertain the needs of children and to outline a course of action best suited for meeting their needs. It is a valuable adjunct for anyone who expects to plan and conduct physical education experiences.

325. Ewing, Neil. GAMES, STUNTS, AND EXERCISES: A PHYSICAL EDUCATION HANDBOOK FOR ELEMENTARY SCHOOL TEACHERS. Fearon-Pitman, Belmont, Calif. 1964.

326. Figley, Grace E.; Mitchell, Heidie; and Wright, Barbara. ELEMENTARY SCHOOL PHYSICAL EDUCATION: AN EDUCATIONAL EXPERIENCE. Kendall-Hunt, Dubuque, Iowa. 1977.

327. Lyttle, Richard B. THE COMPLETE BEGINNER'S GUIDE TO
     PHYSICAL FITNESS (Gr. 1, up). Doubleday, New York.
     1978.

328. Lyttle, Richard B. JOGGING AND RUNNING (Gr. 5, up).
     Watts, New York. 1979.

329. Prudden, Bonnie. FITNESS FROM SIX TO TWELVE. Harper
     & Row, New York. 1972.

330. Prudden, Bonnie. HOW TO KEEP YOUR CHILD FIT FROM BIRTH
     TO SIX. Harper & Row, New York. 1964.

331. Prudden, Bonnie. TEENAGE FITNESS. Harper & Row, New
     York. 1965.

     Exercises and programs described in this book aid teen-
     agers in preparing for sports such as skiing, rock
     climbing, swimming, tumbling, and others. It begins
     with a self-test for fitness and gives very good
     description and treatment for injuries.

332. Prudden, Suzy, and Sussman, Jeffrey. SUZY PRUDDEN'S
     FAMILY FITNESS BOOK. Grosset & Dunlap, New York. 1978.

333. Teodorescu, Redu, and Roberts, Brooks. KID FITNESS.
     Seaview Books, New York. 1979.

     This complete book of fitness exercises for children has
     198 different exercises, all accompanied by handsome,
     clear photographs. Suitable exercises are offered for
     children ranging in age from a few months to 11 years.

334. Walsh, John. FIRST BOOK OF PHYSICAL FITNESS (Gr. 4 - 6).
     Watts, New York. 1961.

Karate, Judo, and T'ai Chi

335. Adams, Brian. MEDICAL IMPLICATIONS OF KARATE BLOWS. Barnes, Cranbury, N.J. 1978.

336. Arneil, Steve, and Dowler, Bryan. BETTER KARATE: THE KEYS TO BETTER TECHNIQUE. New ed. Soccer, New Rochelle, N.Y. 1976.

337. Bartlett, E. G. BASIC JUDO. Arco, New York. 1975.

This book studies the basic principles of judo in particular the techniques of falling, the forty basic throws, the system (The Gokyo), groundwork movements, and three of the Katas or formal demonstrations of the art.

338. Bartlett, E. G. JUDO AND SELF-DEFENSE. Arc Books, New York. 1971.

This book contains 100 carefully graduated lessons in judo and self-defense. Lessons on theory required for each of the grading examinations up to Black Belt 1st Dan of the main judo associations in Great Britain are followed by material on such subjects as continuous attack, counter movements, standing defenses, and self-defense.

339. Bruce, Jeannette. JUDO: A GENTLE BEGINNING. T.Y. Crowell, New York. 1975.

Clever stories and illustrations enhance this excellent book on judo for children. The author skillfully describes the history, physical preparation, lessons on breakfalls, balance throwing, and planning techniques.

340. Burns, Donald J. AN INTRODUCTION TO KARATE FOR STUDENT AND TEACHER. Kendall-Hunt, Dubuque, Iowa. 1977.

341. Cheng Man-Ch'ing, and Smith, Robert W. T'AI-CHI. Charles E. Tuttle Co., Rutland, Vt. 1966.

The authors, masters of the martial arts of the Orient, introduce the reader to T'ai Chi for health, sport, and self-defense and communicate the philosophy inherent in

the practice of this ancient Taoist art. The book
provides step-by-step directions with 275 photographs
of Cheng's 37 solo exercise postures, 122 food weight-
ing diagrams, and a fold-out diagram of postures. This
highly recommended book also contains excellent chapters on Yang Cheng-Fu (Professor Cheng's teacher),
T'ai Chi history and T'ai Chi Ch'uan classics.

342. Chow, David, and Spangler, Richard. KUNG FU: HISTORY,
     PHILOSOPHY, AND TECHNIQUE. Doubleday, New York. 1977.

In response to hundreds of thousands of requests for
information about the show "Kung Fu," the technical
advisory office of Warner Brothers Studio felt an obli-
gation to write their interpretation of the evolution
and philosophy of this ancient Chinese unarmed fighting
system. The authors probe the realities behind some of
the enigmas, and examine the obscure and sometimes
weighty history of the Chinese martial arts along with
a fascinating discussion of techniques and styles of
Kung Fu.

343. Dobson, Terry, and Miller, Victor. GIVING IN TO GET
     YOUR WAY. Delacorte, New York. 1978.

This fascinating and unique book is about Altach-Tics,
the system which combines the martial arts of Aikido
and the rehearsal and training process of the theater.
Altach-Tics uses the physical throws and body movements
of Aikido as metaphors for ways to handle forms of
social or psychological attack.

344. Egami, Shigeru. THE WAY OF KARATE: BEYOND TECHNIQUE.
     Kodansha International, New York. 1976.

This large, fully illustrated book on karate written by
the president and chief instructor of the Shoto-kan of
the Japan Karate-do Shoto-kai delves deeply into the
development of man's spiritual and physical nature.
The beginner can learn the basic skills and develop
the discipline that checks the misuse of such skills.

345. Frommer, Harvey. THE MARTIAL ARTS: JUDO AND KARATE. Atheneum, New York. 1978.

This book presents an overview of the basics of judo and karate. It is a good starting point for anyone interested in the Eastern martial arts. The author discusses the participation in the martial arts of such celebrities as Ryan O'Neal, Steve McQueen, James Cann, Peter Fonda, Herb Alpert, James Coburn, Robert Goulet, and Mike Connors.

346. Gleason, G. R. BETTER JUDO. Rev. ed. Soccer, New Rochelle, N.Y. 1978.

The author treats judo as a sport and not as street fighting and presents illustrated, easy-to-follow exercises and movements in this light.

347. Goldstein, Frances. KARATE FOR KIDS. Arco, New York. 1977.

The author attempts to make this excellently illustrated book simulate the experience gained from discipline exercised in the dajo or training hall. The most effective style of karate practice and defense are combined so that going through complete exercise twice a week will result in beneficial training.

348. Gwon, Pu G. DYNAMIC ART OF BREAKING. Wehman, Cedar Knolls, N.J. 1977.

349. Haines, Bruce. KARATE'S HISTORY AND TRADITIONS. Charles E. Tuttle Co., Rutland, Vt. 1968.

The author writes expressly to counteract the Western trend toward misinformation about Asian martial arts. He offers the reader a well-documented book about Asian history, the origin of karate, and the close connection with Zen Buddhism.

350. Harrington, A. P. DEFEND YOURSELF WITH KUNG FU: A PRACTICAL GUIDE. Barnes & Noble Books, New York. 1977.

351. Huang, Wen-Shan. FUNDAMENTALS OF T'AI CHI CH'UAN.
     South Sky Book Co., New York. 1973.

     This book includes translations of some of the most
     important classics on T'ai Chi and presents an exposi-
     tion of the history, philosophy, technique, practice,
     and fundamentals of the art. The principles of both
     Chinese philosophy and Oriental medicine are incorpor-
     ated into the text, and a section devoted to technical
     directions for the postures is illustrated with photo-
     graphs.

352. James, Stuart. THE COMPLETE BEGINNER'S GUIDE TO JUDO.
     Doubleday, New York. 1978.

353. Kauz, Herman. T'AI CHI HANDBOOK. Doubleday & Co.,
     New York. 1974.

     The author, who has spent most of his life studying the
     martial arts of the East, has written a book considered
     to be the best exercise manual on T'ai Chi. The pos-
     tures are explained and demonstrated in large, clear
     photographs, and material is included on T'ai Chi as a
     meditational technique.

354. Kimmelman, Susan, and Horwitz, Tem, eds. TAI CHI
     CHUAN. Chicago Review, Chicago. 1977.

355. King, Richard A. THE KARATE CONSCIOUSNESS. Ascension,
     Alexandria, Virginia. 1978.

356. Kozuki, Russell. KARATE FOR YOUNG PEOPLE. Corner-
     stone Library, New York. 1975.

357. Lee, Bruce. BRUCE LEE'S FIGHTING METHOD. Wehman,
     Cedar Knolls, N.J. 1977.

358. Lee, Bruce, and Uyehara, M. BRUCE LEE'S FIGHTING
     METHOD. Ohara Publications, Burbank, Calif. 1978.

     Bruce Lee suffered sudden death at age 32. Now his
     friend, Uyehara, has compiled this book which is amply
     illustrated with photographs chosen from among thou-
     sands in Lee's personal photographic file. Lee

combined the knowledge of martial arts expertise with
acting skills and cinematic techniques.

359. Liang, T. T. T'AI CHI CH'UAN FOR HEALTH AND SELF-
     DEFENSE: PHILOSOPHY AND PRACTICE. Random House, New
     York. 1977.

360. Mart, Harry. KUNG FU BIBLE. Atlantis-by-the-Sea,
     New York. 1979.

361. Minick, Michael. KUNG FU: HEALTH SECRETS OF ANCIENT
     CHINA. Simon & Schuster, New York. 1974.

     This book on Kung Fu provides the reader with a fascin-
     ating glimpse into a world of physical therapy that
     Western science has just begun to explore. The system
     described in this book is more than just a pattern of
     exercises; it is an integral part of Chinese medicine.

362. Morris, P. M. THE ILLUSTRATED GUIDE TO KARATE.
     Van Nostrand Reinhold, New York. 1979.

363. Nakayama, Masatoshi. BEST KARATE. (Series 1 to 5).
     Kodansha, New York. 1978.

     The author systematically arranges the basic steps for
     learning karate. He describes the parts of the body
     used as natural weapons, the stances, how to block, how
     to attack, and introduces the reader to the Kata and to
     Kumite. The fundamentals presented in this volume are
     based on the author's 46 years of experience in the art
     of self-defense and on the empirical findings of recent
     research.

364. Nicol, C. W. MOVING ZEN: KARATE AS A WAY TO GENTLENESS.
     Morrow, New York. 1975.

     This book concerns the author's personal experiences
     and travels in pursuing the discipline and rewards of
     karate.

365. Neff, Fred. KARATE IS FOR ME. Lerner Publications,
     Minneapolis. 1979.

366. Nishioka, Hayward. THE JUDO TEXTBOOK. Ohara Publica-
     tions, New York. 1979.

367. Oyama, Mas. MAS OYAMA'S ESSENTIAL KARATE. Ohara
     Publications, New York. 1979.

     This method of nonviolent karate, developed by the
     author, emphasizes the mental and physical states of
     awareness and alertness at all times. The book de-
     scribes the techniques punch-by-punch and kick-by-kick.
     Explicit photographs are included.

368. Reay, Tony, and Hobbs, Geoffrey. THE ILLUSTRATED GUIDE
     TO JUDO. Van Nostrand Reinhold, New York. 1979.

     This all-encompassing book, in a large-sized paperback
     format, covers not only exercises and training programs
     but also areas of health and diet which are so essential
     in perfecting judo techniques. The authors, in addition
     to requisite first steps to be taken in approaching judo,
     also present material covering throws, groundwork, and
     contests.

369. Russel, W. Scott. KARATE: THE ENERGY CONNECTION.
     Delacorte, New York. 1976.

370. Sampayo, Carlos. KARATE WITHIN YOUR GRASP. Sterling,
     New York. 1976.

     Clearly illustrated, this small volume describes how to
     prepare one's body for the systemic, practical exercises
     which will enable one to master karate. Pointing out
     that tremendous amounts of energy are used in karate
     training, the author emphasizes the need for proper food
     and diet and provides essential information thereon.

371. Savai, Kenichi. THE ESSENCE OF KUNG-FU. Japan
     Publications, New York. 1976.

372. Scott, William. CHINESE KUNG FU. Wehman, Cedar Knolls,
     N.J. 1976.

373. Soo, Clifford C. KUNG FU FOR GIRLS AND WOMEN. Gordon-
     Cremonesi, New York. 1979.

374. Tegner, Bruce. BRUCE TEGNER'S COMPLETE BOOK OF JUDO.
     Rev. ed. Thor, Ventura, Calif. 1975.

     This overview of judo describes techniques which apply
     to modern contest and to traditional formal judo. The
     author, whose parents were professional teachers of
     judo and jujitsu, is regarded as an outstanding
     authority, teacher, and innovator in the field.

375. Yang, Ming-Shih. ILLUSTRATED T'AI CHI CH'UAN FOR
     HEALTH AND BEAUTY. Japan Publications, New York. 1976.

FOOD AND NUTRITION

Ben Franklin, an early American commentator, wrote,
"In general, mankind, since the improvement of cookery,
eats twice as much as nature requires." Two hundred years
after Mr. Franklin's observation, overconsumption has become a national pasttime. Not only do we eat more than we
require but we eat less of those foods that satisfy basic
nutritional needs. Western societies are rampantly and
ravenously consuming foods of marginal nutritional value.

The food we eat and how we eat it can enhance health
or contribute to illness. Disabling and killing conditions
such as obesity, malnutrition, diabetes, and hypertension
are strongly diet-related. Best-seller lists are laden with
books telling us to eat less and suggesting ways to do it.
Fasting is an old therapeutic technique. People often stop
eating when ill, and abstain from food until health is
restored.

The Hunza people of the Himalayas are considered "the
healthiest people in the world." Researchers attribute
diet as the major factor in their unusual health and longevity. The Hunzas use food as fuel for the body and consume grains, fruits, assorted raw vegetables and drink small
quantities of goat milk.

In contrast, the U.S. Senate reports that overconsumption and undernutrition figure in five of the ten leading
causes of death: diseases of the heart, cerebrovascular
diseases, diabetes mellitus, arteriosclerosis, and cirrhosis
of the liver.

The importance of early attention to diet is reflected
in the number of overweight children who grow up to be about
one-third of the nation's obese adults. Major prevention
efforts are best directed toward the young because obesity
in adults is difficult to control. The statistics are not
only discouraging but staggering: Ninety-five percent of
people who lose weight, gain it back. Moreover, people are
beginning to suffer a first heart attack at an earlier age.

Many socially minded people are concerned with ways to
affect food choices of the young. However complex the

etiology of these decisions, there is little doubt that
family role modeling plays a major role in the food choices
of the young. Parents who learn sound nutrition and healthy
eating practices will most likely be able by example to
teach their offspring choices to deal successfully with
that ubiquitous and demanding occupation: eating.

FOOD AND NUTRITION

General

376. Airola, Paavo. **ARE YOU CONFUSED?** Health Plus
Publications, Phoenix, Arizona. 1971

The author, a world-famous nutritionist and naturo-
pathic doctor, does an excellent job of helping to
"de-confuse" the confused reader about the many questions pertaining to health and, particularly, pertaining
to nutrition. Dr. Airola's book is complete and extremely useful to those in the healing professions as
well as the layperson. Included are discussions on
macrobiotics, fasts, the dry brush massage, water controversies and biological medicine.

377. Arlin, Marion T. THE SCIENCE OF NUTRITION. 2nd ed.
Macmillan, New York. 1977.

This text introduces the science of nutrition to the
reader who desires a general background in the subject.
The author offers some reasons why nutrition is considered a dynamic component of contemporary life affecting personal experience, welfare of the family, and the
fulfillment of humanity's potential.

378. Arnow, E. Earle. FOOD POWER: A DOCTOR'S GUIDE TO
COMMONSENSE NUTRITION. Nelson-Hall, Chicago. 1972.

The author discusses the relationship of biochemistry
and clinical dietetics to the field of nutrition.

379. Ashley, Richard, and Duggal, Heidi. DICTIONARY OF
NUTRITION. Pocket Bks., New York. 1976.

380. Bauer, Cathy, and Anderson, Juel. THE TOFU COOKBOOK.
Rodale Press, Emmaus, Pa. 1979.

381. Bender, A. E. DICTIONARY OF NUTRITION AND FOOD
TECHNOLOGY. Chemical Publications, New York. 1977.

382. Bernard, Raymond. EAT YOUR WAY TO BETTER HEALTH.
Saucerian, Clarksburg, W.Va. 1974.

383. Blaine, Tom R. MENTAL HEALTH THROUGH NUTRITION.
Citadel Press, Secaucus, N.J. 1975.

This book is one of the few books written which relates
mental health to nutrition. It is a down-to-earth study
of how vitamin and mineral deficiencies are responsible
for most of our physical and mental illnesses. Discussions are included as to how proper diet and vitamin
therapy can help cure nervous tension, chronic fatigue,
depression, insomnia, and even schizophrenia.

384. Blaine, Tom R. NUTRITION AND YOUR HEART. Keats,
New Canaan, Conn. 1979.

This book presents a program of natural nutrition that
supplies the elements needed to prevent heart disease.
The author examines vitamins, minerals, foods, exercise,
and dispels medical myths and misconceptions about heart
disease.

385. Bradshaw, Lois, and Mazlen, G. NUTRITION IN HEALTH
CARE. Creative Informatics, Aspen, Colo. 1979.

386. Briggs, George M., and Calloway, Doris H. BOGERT'S
NUTRITION AND PHYSICAL FITNESS. 10th ed. Saunders,
Philadelphia. 1979.

387. Caliendo, Mary A. NUTRITION AND THE WORLD FOOD CRISIS.
Macmillan, New York. 1979.

The contents of this book emphasize the problems and
circumstances that currently afflict Third World nations.
The author discusses factors that influence agriculture,
food production, and food distribution. This book is a
practical resource for teachers and students engaged in
any aspect of nutrition education.

388. Carque, Otto. VITAL FACTS ABOUT FOODS. Keats, New
Canaan, Conn. 1975.

389. Clark, Linda. HOW TO IMPROVE YOUR HEALTH: THE
     WHOLISTIC APPROACH. Keats, New Canaan, Conn. 1979.

     The author is a reporter who has researched and written
     on many aspects of natural healing and nutrition.   In
     this book, Ms. Clark offers brief but complete descrip-
     tions of various "alternative therapies," including
     color and sound therapies, herbal therapy, osteopathy,
     homeopathy, acupressure, natureopathy, and spiritual
     healing among others.

390. Clark, Linda. KNOW YOUR NUTRITION. (Spanish ed.)
     Keats, New Canaan, Conn. 1979.

391. Clarkson, Kenneth W. FOOD STAMPS AND NUTRITION. AEI
     (American Enterprise Institute for Public Policy
     Research), Washington, D.C. 1975.

     This book measures the two objectives of the food stamp
     program: improving nutrition among the poor and supple-
     menting the low income of farmers. Based on well-
     founded research and analyses, the author explains why
     and how the present program serves neither objective
     well.

392. Clydesdale, Fergus. FOOD SCIENCE AND NUTRITION: CURRENT
     ISSUES AND ANSWERS. Prentice-Hall, Englewood Cliffs,
     N.J. 1978.

393. Creff, Albert, and Wernick, Robert. DR. CREFF'S 1-2-3
     SPORTS DIET. Coward, McCann & Geoghegan, New York.
     1979.

394. Crisp, Arthur H., and Stonehill, Edward. SLEEP,
     NUTRITION AND MOOD. Wiley Intl., New York. 1976.

     This monograph attempts to clarify some of the clinical
     links between sleep, activity, nutrition, and mood pat-
     terns. The authors, who are clinical psychiatrists,
     show particular interest in subjects affected with
     primary anorexia nervosa and examine the quantification
     of some of the aspects of these basic problems.

395. Darden, Ellington. NUTRITION FOR ATHLETES. Anna
     Publications, Winter Park, Florida. 1978.

     This book exposes many of the myths that surround nutri-
     tion in the sports world and provides easy-to-understand
     guidelines for improved athletic performance.

396. D'Asaro, Barbara. BE YOUNG AND VITAL: THE NUTRITION
     EXERCISE PLAN. Enslow, Short Hills, N.J. 1979.

397. Dean, Margaret C. THE COMPLETE GOURMET NUTRITION
     COOKBOOK. Acropolis Books Ltd., Washington, D.C. 1980.

     The author, a noted nutritionist, combines advice and
     recipes to help everyone onto the healthy road to eat-
     ing well and right. She has put the complex findings
     of the U. S. Senate Select Committee on Nutrition and
     Human Needs into 581 easy-to-prepare and delicious
     recipes and menus. The book contains chapters with
     nutritional advice on many problems that plague modern
     life: weight control, inflation, stress, changing life-
     styles, special dietary diseases, and our loss of en-
     joyment in eating.

398. Deatherage, F. E. FOOD FOR LIFE. Plenum, New York.
     1975.

     Everything concerning food is described in depth in this
     book: how food is produced, processed, distributed and
     consumed; problems of spoilage and preservation; food
     components; the digestive process; and world population
     growth and future food supplies. The author attempts
     to present an integrated view of the physical, bio-
     logical, and social sciences of food for peoples of the
     world. Governmental regulation of food, consumer pro-
     tection, regulatory agencies, and the role of government
     in the control of international commerce are also re-
     viewed. The text is intended for university students,
     professionals, and the general reader.

399. Deutsch, Ronald M. THE NEW NUTS AMONG THE BERRIES.
     Bull, Palo Alto, Calif. 1977.

     This delightful, imaginative book discusses the capitula-
     tion of prominent American figures to the sirens of

nutrition nonsense. The author candidly discusses the
nutrition experts themselves and the diets they propose.

400. DeVore, Sally, and White, Thelma. DINNER'S READY! AN
     INVITATION TO BETTER NUTRITION FROM NINE HEALTHIER
     SOCIETIES. Doubleday, New York. 1978.

The authors discuss the fascinating nutritional back-
grounds and recipes of different peoples (Hunza,
Marquesans, Tuareys of the Sahara, Eskimo, and others)
and conclude with a look at the healthy cultures in the
United States and a general review of the science of
nutrition.

401. Doyle, Rodger P., and Redding, James L. THE COMPLETE
     FOOD HANDBOOK: THE NINETEEN EIGHTY EDITION. Grove,
     New York. 1979.

This clearly written volume examines the nutritional
value and the safety of additives of many products sold
in supermarkets and health food stores. The book gives
the reader an informative overview of the food industry
and deals with the dangers of environmental contaminants
and the fraudulent claims of health faddists.

402. Echols, Barbara E., and Arena, Jay M. THE COMMON-SENSE
     GUIDE TO GOOD EATING. Barron Educational Bks., Woodbury,
     N.J. 1978.

The authors outline five essential requirements for
sensible weight control and good eating habits and
consider the practice of vegetarianism and the use of
health foods as alternative ways to traditional eating.
How to lose, gain, or maintain weight, and other common
issues and problems of nutrition today are examined.

403. Ewart, Charles D. HOW TO ENJOY EATING WITHOUT
     COMMITTING SUICIDE. Cornerstone Library, New York. 1973.

The author's background of over 20 years in the market-
ing of food products and his ability to simplify complicated subjects enables him to write this concise,
practical guide on the fundamentals of nutrition in

non-scientific language. This book also shows the
reader how to benefit from the latest government label-
ing regulations.

404. Feinman, Jeffrey. CATALOG OF FOOD. Doubleday, New
York. 1977.

This catalog of fine edibles and kitchen equipment
describes the most exciting, freshest, and exotic kinds
of foods and tells where to get them. Enhanced with
over 300 illustrations, this guide allows the reader to
shop for gourmet foods, health and organic foods, international groceries, freeze-dried camping foods, and unusual kitchen utensils.

405. Ferguson, James M., and Taylor, C. Barr. A CHANGE FOR
HEART: YOUR FAMILY AND THE FOOD YOU EAT. Bull, Palo
Alto, Calif. 1978.

406. Fisher, Patty, and Bender, Arnold E. THE VALUE OF FOOD.
2nd ed. Oxford Univ. Press, New York. 1975.

407. Fleming, June. THE WELL-FED BACKPACKER. Victoria
House, Portland, Oregon. 1979.

This excellent handbook, written by an experienced backpacker, covers everything the outdoors person would need
to know about food preparation. Packaging, emergency
food, dried and wild foods are just a few of the topics
discussed.

408. Ford, Norman D. GOOD HEALTH WITHOUT DRUGS: GET WELL
AND STAY WELL THE NATURAL WAY. St. Martin's Press,
New York. 1978.

409. Fredericks, Carlton. CARLTON FREDERICKS' HIGH FIBER WAY
TO TOTAL HEALTH. Pocket Books, New York. 1976.

President of the International Academy of Preventive
Medicine, Fredericks is a leader in the avant garde
nutrition field. The author feels that problems such
as bowel cancer, appendicitis, diverticular disease,
hemorrhoids and varicose veins can be cured or prevented
through a high fiber diet. The book is an excellent
source for benefits and misconceptions about fiber.

410. Fredericks, Carlton. PSYCHO-NUTRITION. Grosset & Dunlap, New York. 1976.

This book focuses on megavitamins and orthomolecular therapy. The author is a well-known nutritionist who discusses hypoglycemia, schizophrenia, autism, allergies, and a whole range of chemical malfunctions. He provides case histories and research findings and includes an appendix on where to seek help.

411. Fredericks, Carlton, and Bailey, Herbert. FOOD FACTS AND FALLACIES. Arc Books, New York. 1968.

Carlton Fredericks' name is a household word in public health education, having taught nutrition at several universities and on the radio for many years. The author's anti-establishment views are eminently sound; but, where needed, he is critical of health foods and fads. This book covers a cornucopia of subjects: diet supplements, fluoridation, various diseases, aging, mental illness, sex and diet, weight, the FDA and AMA, and much more.

412. Gallender, Carolyn N., and Gallender, Demos. DIETARY PROBLEMS AND DIETS FOR THE HANDICAPPED. Charles C Thomas, Springfield, Ill. 1979.

413. Garard, Ira. THE STORY OF FOOD. Avi, Westport, Conn. 1974.

This book of historical anecdotes charts changes in the sources of the food supply from its primitive past to its sophisticated present. The author explains the processing of some of the more important foods, discusses the difficulties of the legal regulation of food, and examines the chemical nature of food and digestion.

414. Gazella, Jacqueline G. NUTRITION FOR THE CHILDBEARING YEAR. Woodland, Wayzata, Minn. 1979.

415. Gerrard, Don. ONE BOWL: A SIMPLE CONCEPT FOR CONTROLLING BODY WEIGHT. Random House, New York. 1974.

416. Goulart, Frances S. EATING TO WIN. Stein & Day,
     Briarcliff Manor, N.Y. 1978.

     This book attempts to relate the value of food to im-
     proved performance in tennis, swimming, cycling, jog-
     ging, handball, skiing, and other sports. The author
     assesses the effects of high protein diets, vegetarian-
     ism, fasting, megavitamins, and nucleic acid diets on
     athletic performance.

417. Grant, Doris. RECIPE FOR SURVIVAL: YOUR DAILY FOOD.
     Keats, New Canaan, Conn. 1974.

     Ms. Grant presents effective and interesting data on the
     value of unprocessed whole grain bread. By exploring
     contaminants in our water, soil, and food, the author
     shows the relationship of present-day eating habits to
     modern diseases. She tells the consumer why products
     such as cooking utensils, detergents, drugs, and H_2O
     softeners pose health problems.

418. Gullet, Jane F. EVERYONE'S GUIDE TO FOOD SELF-
     SUFFICIENCY. Naturegraph, Happy Camp, Calif. 1979

419. Guthrie, Helen. INTRODUCTORY NUTRITION. 4th ed.
     Mosby, St. Louis, Mo. 1979.

     The aim of this book is to help readers discriminate
     between fact and fallacy in the nutritional field and
     to discriminate between scientific and pseudoscientific
     information. Intended for a new kind of student enter-
     ing college with no science training but with a serious
     interest in nutrition, the book contains information
     about fats, proteins, and carbohydrates, and covers
     topics of applied nutrition such as pregnancy, aging,
     and weight control. Included are tables of food compo-
     sition, a glossary of terms, and tables of desirable
     weights for children and adults.

420. Hall, Ross H. FOOD FOR NAUGHT: THE DECLINE IN
     NUTRITION. Random House, New York. 1976.

     A biochemist attacks the increased use of chemicals to
     produce larger crops, fatter livestock, and better
     textured, tenderer food, not because the chemicals are

dangerous in themselves but because they destroy basic
nutritional value. Written for persons with a non-
technical background, the book aims to make readers
aware of the quality of "urbanized" nourishment. Included in an appendix are technical details drawn from
a variety of source material, including technical trade
journals.

421. Halpern, Seymour, ed. QUICK REFERENCE TO CLINICAL
NUTRITION. Lippincott, New York. 1979.

This publication is for the busy physician who needs
updated information about nutrition and metabolism for
use in daily medical practice but does not have time to
become expert. It is not an encyclopedia but rather
emphasizes clinically significant data. Contributors
include specialists in medicine, neurology, surgery,
and pediatrics.

422. Hamilton, Eva M., and Whitney, Eleanor N. NUTRITION:
CONCEPTS AND CONTROVERSY. West Publishing, St. Paul,
Minn. 1979.

Scientific principles of nutrition, guidelines for food
choices, and techniques for meeting the challenge of the
information explosion are presented in this excellent
text for the concerned consumer. The authors present
solid evidence for and against current "hot topics" in
nutrition such as the FDA, Vitamin E, saccharin, and
the world food crisis.

423. Hansen, R. Gaurth, and Wyse, Bonita W. NUTRITIONAL
INDEX OF FOOD QUALITY. Avi, Westport, Conn. 1979.

424. Hatfield, Antoinette K., and Stanton, Peggy S. HOW TO
HELP YOUR CHILD EAT RIGHT: A FUN COOKBOOK AND GUIDE TO
GOOD NUTRITION. Acropolis, Washington, D.C. 1978.

This book stresses the need for creativity in nutrition
education and encourages mothers to promote the principles of good nutrition especially during the rapid-
growth period of children.

425. Hegne, Barbara. EVERYWOMAN'S EVERY DAY EXERCISE AND
NUTRITION BOOK. Keats, New Canaan, Conn. 1979.

426. Hightower, Jim. EAT YOUR HEART OUT. Vintage/Random
House, New York. 1976.

This technical but interesting book reveals the un-
scrupulous tactics used by huge conglomerates to control
the price and quality of the food we buy. The author
documents the reasons why costs and profits are spiral-
ing everupward.

427. Hofmann, Lieselotte. THE GREAT AMERICAN NUTRITION
HASSLE. Mayfield, Palo Alto, Calif. 1978.

Various experts contribute views on nutritional attitudes, needs, and hazards, for example: the psychology
and physiology of eating; the dangers of alcohol, drugs,
sugar, and cholesterol; and food additives.

428. Hunter, Beatrice T. THE GREAT NUTRITION ROBBERY.
Scribner, New York. 1978.

429. Jacobson, Michael F. NUTRITION SCOREBOARD. Avon,
New York. 1979.

This practical guide rates the nutritional value of food
and includes a scoring device for estimating vitamin and
mineral content. Scoreboards are presented on soups,
breads, frozen meals, snacks, desserts, and breakfast
foods, as well as a quiz for rating your own diet.
Special sections are devoted to food additives, the
cholesterol question, calories, salt, and alcohol.

430. Jordan, Henry; Levitz, Leonard S.; and Kimbrell, Gordon
M. EATING IS OKAY: A RADICAL APPROACH TO WEIGHT LOSS.
New American Library, New York. 1978.

431. Katch, Frank I., and McArdle, William D. NUTRITION,
WEIGHT CONTROL AND EXERCISE. Houghton Mifflin, Boston.
1977.

432. Kaufman, William I. GUIDE TO CALORIES. Baronet, New
York. 1978.

433. Kaufman, William I. GUIDE TO CARBOHYDRATES. Baronet,
     New York. 1978.

     What are carbohydrates and how does a low-carbohydrate
     diet differ from a calorie-counting diet? Answers to
     these and other questions are provided in this complete
     guide to carbohydrates which also includes menus,
     recipes, and special diet tips. Included are tables of
     carbohydrate content of approximately 1,000 basic foods
     based on information from the U. S. Department of
     Agriculture.

434. Kaufman, William I. GUIDE TO CHOLESTEROL. Baronet,
     New York. 1978.

435. Kaufman, William I. GUIDE TO PROTEINS. Baronet, New
     York. 1978.

436. Kaysing, Bill. EAT WELL ON A DOLLAR A DAY. Chronicle
     Books, San Francisco. 1975.

437. Kirschmann, John D., ed. NUTRITION ALMANAC. Rev. ed.
     McGraw-Hill, New York. 1979.

     This almanac is a useful tool for the reader who wants
     to work out a total plan for personal nutrition and who
     wants answers to some simple questions about food,
     nutrition, and health.

438. Kordel, Lelord. YOU'RE YOUNGER THAN YOU THINK. Popular
     Library, New York. 1979.

439. Kowalski, Gene. HOW TO EAT CHEAP BUT GOOD. Popular
     Library, New York. 1977.

440. Kowtaluk, Helen, and Kopan, Alice. FOOD FOR TODAY.
     C. A. Bennett, Peoria, Ill. 1977.

441. Kraus, Barbara. UNITED NATIONS COOKBOOK. Simon &
     Schuster, New York. 1970.

     These recipes from all over the world represent the best
     selection of native dishes from all 126 member nations
     of the U. N.

442. Kretchmer, Norman, and Robertson, William Van B.
     HUMAN NUTRITION. Scientific American. W. H. Freeman
     & Co., San Francisco. 1978.

443. Labuza, T. P., and Sloan, A. Elizabeth.   FOOD FOR
     THOUGHT. 2nd ed. Avi, Westport, Conn. 1977.

     This overview of nutritional concepts and food science
     theories provides the novitiate with the knowledge to
     make sound judgments about the quality or usefulness of
     a particular food. The authors feel that these judg-
     ments can best be accomplished by learning about the
     interactions of food components during digestion and
     knowing the chemical needs of the body. The authors
     evaluate the effects of processing on nutritional value
     and the safety of food additives.

444. Lansky, Vicki. THE TAMING OF THE C.A.N.D.Y. MONSTER.
     Meadowbrook Press, Wayzata, Minn. 1978.

445. Lappe, Frances M., and Collins, Joseph. FOOD FIRST: BE-
     YOND THE MYTH OF SCARCITY. Houghton Mifflin, Boston. 1977.

     This book is written in a question and answer format.
     The authors tackle certain food assumptions and demon-
     strate how these have actually impeded efforts to end
     starvation. The questions focus around the themes of
     overpopulation, pro's and con's of mechanized farming,
     pesticides, and the "green revolution" relative to
     famine in India and Africa. Ms. Lappe, one of the
     authors of this book, wrote the well-known Diet for a
     Small Planet (Ballantine, New York. 1975).

446. Larsen, Egon. FOOD: PAST, PRESENT AND FUTURE. Crane-
     Russak Co., New York. 1978.

447. Lasota, Marcia. THE FAST FOOD CALORIE GUIDE. Minnesota
     Scholarly Press, Mankato, Minn. 1979.

448. Lesser, Michael. NUTRITION AND VITAMIN THERAPY. Grove,
     New York. 1979.

     This book on preventive medicine demonstrates the con-
     nection between poor nutritional habits and environment-
     al pollutants to the resulting imbalances in the body.

The author describes the vital components of body chemistry explaining each of the vitamins and minerals in
layman's terms, and devotes special chapters to the role
nutrition plays in allergies, blood sugar levels, mental
and emotional disturbances, and sexual vitality.

449. Lewin, Brenda. SENSUOUS NUTRITION. Major Books, Canoga
     Park, Calif. 1977.

450. Lewis, Christine. THE FOOD CHOICE JUNGLE. Merrimack
     Book Service, Bridgeport, Conn. 1979.

The author explains the reasons food choice relates to
health and well-being. Parents of young children will
learn how to provide food for optimum health and begin
good food habits that can last a lifetime. The book
assists homemakers with shopping lists and menu planning,
instructs the reader in balancing the diet and budget,
and helps the elderly know which basic foods to choose.

451. Lief, Stanley. HOW TO EAT FOR HEALTH. Baronet, New
     York. 1979.

452. Loewenfeld, Claire. EVERYTHING YOU SHOULD KNOW ABOUT
     YOUR FOOD. Merrimack Book Service, Bridgeport, Conn.
     1978.

This informative book written by a strong supporter of a
more self-sufficient lifestyle, points out the content
and disadvantages of refined and convenience foods and
underlines the advantages of naturally balanced and un-
processed foods.

The author's experience in organic gardening, herbal use
and nutrition offers a wealth of information, including
at-a-glance nutrition charts, home preserving, meal
planning, cooking with herbs, specialized needs of select populations, and the importance of food education.

453. Lowenberg, Miriam E.; Todhunter, Neige; Wilson, Eva;
     Feeny, Moira C.; and Savage, Jan R. FOOD AND PEOPLE.
     3rd ed. Wiley Intl., New York. 1979.

454. Luna, David. FITNESS AND THE SENSIBLE DIET. Peace
     Press, Culver City, Calif. 1980.

455. MacAdie, Diana. HEALTHY EATING. Merrimack Book
     Service, Bridgeport, Conn. 1978.

     A concise, clearly written book on nutritional needs,
     diets of different population groups, alternative diets,
     along with a basic description of minerals, vitamins,
     and protein.

456. Margolese, Richard G. DOCTOR'S EAT-HEARTY GUIDE FOR
     GOOD HEALTH AND LONG LIFE. Prentice-Hall, Englewood
     Cliffs, N.J. 1974.

457. Mayer, Jean. A DIET FOR LIVING. Pocket Books, New
     York, 1976.

     The author's reverence for good food and hearty appe-
     tites is tempered by Mayer's dismay at the enormous
     quantities of bad food consumed. The nation's foremost
     authority on nutrition and health tells the reader all
     about food and the heart, food sources for vitamins and
     minerals, overweight, underweight, and much more.

458. Mayer, Jean. HUMAN NUTRITION: ITS PHYSIOLOGICAL,
     MEDICAL AND SOCIAL ASPECTS. Charles C Thomas, Spring-
     field, Ill. 1979.

     An all-inclusive tome, this book discusses the scientif-
     ic, clinical, and administrative aspects of nutrition in
     relation to health, poverty, war, and technology.
     Eighty-two essays cover all aspects of nutrition--psycho-
     logical, medical, and social--and discuss such topics as
     calories and the need for energy, the need for nutrients,
     the seven ages of man from infancy to old age, hunger
     and obesity, inborn errors of metabolism, nutrition and
     disease, safety of foods, dietetics, and nutrition and
     the world. Very complete food composition tables are
     included.

459. McGraw-Hill Editors. MCGRAW-HILL ENCYCLOPEDIA OF FOOD,
     AGRICULTURE, AND NUTRITION. McGraw-Hill, New York. 1977.

460. McWilliams, Margaret. FOOD FUNDAMENTALS. 3rd ed.
     Wiley Intl., New York. 1979.

461. Miller, Fred. PASSPORT TO BETTER LIVING THROUGH EATING.
Aztex, Tucson, Arizona. 1979.

462. Moyer, Ann. THE FIBER FACTOR. Rodale Press, Emmaus,
Pa. 1976.

This book is intended to advise the reader what bran can
and cannot do; how the addition to the diet of food
fiber can help the reader from falling victim to the
diseases of civilization, constipation, hemorrhoids,
varicose veins, and others. Included is an excellent
description of what actually happens inside the digestive tract and circulatory system when disease strikes
and just how bran works to solve these problems.

463. Moyer, Ann. BETTER FOOD FOR PUBLIC PLACES - A GUIDE FOR
IMPROVING INSTITUTIONAL FOOD. Rodale Press, Emmaus, Pa.
1977.

464. Mulhauser, Roland. MORE VITAMINS AND MINERALS WITH
FEWER CALORIES. C. E. Tuttle, Rutland, Vt. 1978.

465. Nichols, Joe D., and Presley, James. PLEASE DOCTOR, DO
SOMETHING: A MODERN PHYSICIAN LOOKS AT NUTRITION. Devin-
Adair, Old Greenwich, Conn. 1974.

In this lively book, a modern physician uses first-
person stories to look at nutrition and health. Dr.
Nichols' book includes everything from how to grow a
garden to advice on baby foods, anorexia, birth defects,
and breastfeeding.

466. Null, Gary, and Null, Steven. HOW TO GET RID OF THE
POISONS IN YOUR BODY. Arco, New York. 1977.

467. Nutrition Foundation. PRESENT KNOWLEDGE IN NUTRITION.
Nutrition Foundation, Washington, D.C. 1976.

Although this book is not to be viewed as a complete
textbook of nutrition, it is excellent as supplementary
reading for students of nutrition and related fields.
It also provides a means for other professionals to keep
abreast of current progress through authoritative reviews of the current literature in the science of nutrition.

468. Ohsawa, George. MACROBIOTICS; AN INVITATION TO HEALTH
     AND HAPPINESS. Japan Publications, New York. 1976.

469. Olson, Robert E., ed. PROTEIN-CALORIE MALNUTRITION.
     Academic Press, New York. 1975.

     The book considers all aspects of protein-calorie mal-
     nutrition (PCM), from molecular biology to epidemiology
     and prevention. It devotes special attention to the
     controversy of protein versus calories in the develop-
     ment and treatment of disease. It also examines the
     mechanisms underlying the synergism between nutrition
     and infection.

470. Peckham, Gladys C.   FOUNDATIONS OF FOOD PREPARATION.
     3rd. ed. Macmillan, New York. 1974.

     This illustrated edition presents the basic principles
     of food preparation enabling first year college students
     to develop high standards of food preparation.

471. Pelstring, Linda, and Hauck, JoAnn. FOODS TO IMPROVE
     YOUR HEALTH. Walker & Co., New York. 1974.

     The right foods can be an effective preventive measure
     against disease, say the authors. What is in foods and
     the good and bad effects different foods may have on
     the body, especially the heart, brain, and lungs are
     discussed. Tables of dietary allowances are presented
     for infants, children, men, women, and for women during
     pregnancy and lactation.

472. Pfeiffer, Carl C., and Banks, Jane. DR. PFEIFFER'S
     NUTRITIONAL GUIDE TO TOTAL HEALTH. Simon & Schuster,
     New York. 1979.

473. Phillips, David A. GUIDEBOOK TO NUTRITIONAL FACTORS
     IN FOODS. Woodbridge, Santa Barbara, Calif. 1979.

474. Posner, Barbara. NUTRITION AND THE ELDERLY. Lexington
     Books, Lexington, Mass. 1979.

475. Reuben, David. EVERYTHING YOU ALWAYS WANTED TO KNOW
     ABOUT NUTRITION. Simon & Schuster, New York. 1978.

     Basic information about vitamins, minerals, fats, carbo-
     hydrates, proteins, and sugars is summarized. The ideal
     diet is spelled out and often-asked questions about
     nutrition are answered. Dr. Reuben addresses special
     notes to the food industry, to the Food and Drug Admin-
     istration, and to his fellow physicians.

476. Roe, Daphne A. CLINICAL NUTRITION FOR THE HEALTH
     SCIENTIST. CRC Press, Boca Raton, Fla. 1979.

477. Roth, June. THE FOOD-DEPRESSION CONNECTION.
     Contemporary Books, Chicago. 1979.

     This practical, down-to-earth book about food allergies
     concentrates on the day-to-day problems of providing
     adequate nutrition while circumventing specific food
     sensitivities.

478. Rubin, C.; Farago, J.; Etra, J.; Stark, R.; and
     Rollert, D. THE JUNK FOOD BOOK. Dell, New York. 1980.

479. Rubinstein, Paul. JUST GOOD FOOD. Scribner, New York.
     1978.

480. Runyan, Thora J. NUTRITION FOR TODAY. Harper & Row,
     New York. 1976.

     This textbook for the beginning student covers a wide
     range of topics from the science of nutrition to its
     status in the world today.

481. Santa Maria, Jack. THE YOGA OF FOOD. Autumn Press,
     Brookline, Mass. 1979.

482. Schwartz, George. FOOD POWER. McGraw-Hill, New York.
     1979.

483. Scrutton, Robert. NATURE'S WAY TO NUTRITION AND
     VIBRANT HEALTH. Neville Spearman, London. 1976.

     This simple guide to better eating provides excellent
     information on natural foods, discusses meditation,

natural treatment of diseases, rheumatism, homeopathy,
and presents some interesting cases.

484. Sheinken, David, and Shachter, Michael. THE FOOD
CONNECTION: HOW THE THINGS YOU EAT AFFECT THE WAY YOU
FEEL. Bobbs-Merrill, Indianapolis, Ind. 1979.

485. Smith, E. W., Jr. DIETER'S CHECKLIST. Doubleday,
New York. 1975.

486. Soup, Stone. THE KITCHEN ALMANAC. Berkley Publications, New York. 1977.

487. Spira, Michael. HOW TO LOSE WEIGHT WITHOUT REALLY
DIETING. Penguin, New York. 1979.

488. Tilden, J. H. FOOD: ITS INFLUENCE AS A FACTOR IN DIS-
EASE AND HEALTH. Rev. Ed. Keats, New Canaan, Conn. 1976.

Dr. Tilden, one of the founders of the natural hygiene
movement, wrote this book in the early part of the
twentieth century to educate people in the proper food
combinations and to the consumption of unrefined, pure
foods. The language is archaic but the ideas are
modern.

489. Trillin, Calvin. ALICE, LET'S EAT: FURTHER ADVENTURES
OF A HAPPY EATER. Random House, New York. 1979.

490. Vail, Gladys E.; Justin, Margaret M.; and Rust, Lucille
Osborn. FOODS. 7th ed. Houghton Mifflin, Boston. 1978.

491. Verrett, Jacqueline, and Carper, Jean. EATING MAY BE
HAZARDOUS TO YOUR HEALTH. Simon & Schuster, New York.
1974.

The authors alert the consumer to the chemicalization of
food and the government's failure to do something about
it. The authors of this excellent, informative book
are, respectively, a biochemist who was a researcher
with the FDA for 15 years and a consumer-science writer.

492. Wade, Carlson. FACT-BOOK ON HYPERTENSION, HIGH BLOOD
PRESSURE AND YOUR DIET. Keats, New Canaan, Conn. 1975.

493. Wade, Jean G., and Hosier, Helen K. EATING YOUR WAY TO
GOOD HEALTH: THE BIBLE, FOOD AND YOU. Revell, Old
Tappan, N.J. 1977.

A nutritionist looks to passages in the Bible as guidelines to help us choose food wisely. The book includes
chapters on foods in the Bible, vitaminizing and miner-
alizing your body, and types and methods of fasting.

494. Walcher, Dwain N.; Barnett, H. D.; and Kretchmer, N.,
eds. FOOD, MAN AND SOCIETY. New ed. Plenum, New York.
1976.

495. Walczak, Michael, and Ehrich, Benjamin B. NUTRITION AND
WELL-BEING. Mojave Books, Reseda, Calif. 1977.

Writing in a clear direct manner, the author attempts to
bridge the ever-increasing gap in communication between
the lab and the layperson. He shares with the reader
some of his international experiences based on current
medical and biochemical knowledge in the field of nutrition. The book stresses two important points: everyone's biochemical difference and the human system's
struggle for balance.

496. Watson, George. THE PSYCHOCHEMICAL RESPONSE. Harper &
Row, New York. 1979.

497. White, Philip, and Selvey, Nancy, eds. LET'S TALK ABOUT
FOOD. PSG Publishers, Littleton, Mass. 1974.

498. Williams, Roger J. NUTRITION AGAINST DISEASE. Bantam
Books, New York. 1973.

The fundamental premise of this book is based on the
crucially important effects that the microenvironment
of body cells has on health, and that deficiencies in
this environment constitute a major cause of disease.
The author, known as the father of nutrition, writes
about the serious deficiencies in present-day medical
education and supports his findings with a lifetime of
scientific inquiry.

499. Yudkin, John. THIS NUTRITION BUSINESS. St. Martin's,
New York. 1978.

500. Zebroff, Kareen. YOGA AND NUTRITION. Arco, New York.
      1979.

Vegetarianism

501. Altman, Nathaniel. EATING FOR LIFE. Theosophical
Publishing House, Wheaton, Ill. 1977.

A scientific, objective, moral, and humane approach to
vegetarianism, this book offers advice on what to eat
if you do not eat meat and how to save money on a
vegetarian diet. The history of vegetarianism, world
food shortages, ecological considerations of eating
patterns, and vegetarian recipes are also included.

502. Axon, William E. SHELLEY'S VEGETARIANISM. Haskell
House, New York. 1971

503. Bauer, Cathy, and Anderson, Juel. THE TOFU COOKBOOK.
Rodale Press, Emmaus, Pa. 1980.

This cookbook clearly describes how tofu and its by-
products are used in cooking. This no-cholesterol,
high-protein food from the Orient contains only 4% fat,
compared to choice grade hamburger's 25% fat, yet contains comparable protein. Tofu is inexpensive, healthful, and easy to use.

504. Berry, Rynn, Jr. THE VEGETARIANS. Autumn Press,
Brookline, Mass. 1979.

505. Brooks, Karen. FORGET ABOUT MEAT COOKBOOK. Rodale
Press, Emmaus, Pa. 1978.

This unusual book offers recipes and information that
will save food money while adding well-balanced nutrition to your meals. Ms. Brooks, a vegetarian, lived
on an organic farm in Easley, Missouri, where she
farmed and canned most of her food.

506. Chen, Philip S. THE JOY OF BEING A VEGETARIAN. Pacific
Press, Mountain View, Calif. 1977.

The author, an eminent biochemist, heralds the superior-
ity of a vegetable diet. He compares the performance of
vegetarian athletes with that of non-vegetarians and
supports the benefits of vegetable protein by citing information from leaders in the nutrition field.

507. Doyle, Roger. THE VEGETARIAN HANDBOOK. Crown, New York. 1979.

508. Fulton, Alvenia M. VEGETARIAN FACT OR MYTH--EATING TO LIVE. 2nd ed. BCA Publishing, Chicago. 1978.

509. Gay, Kathyln; Gay, Maria; and Gay, Martin. GET HOOKED ON VEGETABLES. (Gr. 7, up) Messner, New York. 1978.

510. Giehl, Dudley. VEGETARIANISM: A WAY OF LIFE. Harper & Row, New York. 1979.

511. Goldstein, Jack. TRIUMPH OVER DISEASE--BY FASTING AND NATURAL DIET. Arco, New York. 1977.

512. Larson, Jeanne, and McLin, Ruth. THE VEGETABLE PROTEIN AND VEGETARIAN COOKBOOK. Arc Books, New York. 1977.

513. Moore, Shirley T., and Byers, Mary P. A VEGETARIAN DIET: WHAT IT IS, HOW TO MAKE IT HEALTHFUL AND ENJOY-ABLE. Woodbridge, Santa Barbara, Calif. 1978.

514. Null, George, and Null, Steve. THE NEW VEGETARIAN. Dell, New York. 1979.

515. Parham, Barbara. WHAT'S WRONG WITH EATING MEAT? Ananda Marga Publ., Denver, Colo. 1979.

There are physiological, ecological, political, moral, and health reasons for not eating meat. This easy-to-read and well-documented book explores each of these areas, giving a well-rounded picture of the universal and widespread sentiment that has led people to vegetarianism, both in the past and present.

516. Shulman, Martha. THE VEGETARIAN FEAST. Harper & Row, New York. 1979.

517. Sussman, Vic. A VEGETARIAN ALTERNATIVE. Rodale Press, Emmaus, Pa. 1978.

A guide to a healthful and humane diet, this book is written in a lively and readable style. It offers good meatless recipes as well as some basic information about how to include proteins, vitamins, and minerals into a

healthful and nutritious diet. The world food crisis
is discussed.

518. Thomas, Anna. THE VEGETARIAN EPICURE. Knopf, New York.
     1978.

519. Whyte, Karen C. THE ORIGINAL DIET, RAW VEGETARIAN GUIDE
     AND RECIPE BOOK. Troubadour Press, San Francisco. 1977.

     The author tells the dramatic story of mankind's dietary
     origins, and attempts to show why a natural raw food
     diet (vegetables, fruit, and nuts) is best. The book
     includes information on where to buy and how to prepare
     and preserve raw foods and presents over 150 ingenious
     and tasty recipes.

520. Zurbel, Victor, and Zurbel, Runa. THE VEGETARIAN
     FAMILY: WITH RECIPES FOR A HEALTHIER LIFE. Prentice-
     Hall, Englewood Cliffs, N.J. 1973.

Weight Loss

521. Bricklin, Mark. LOSE WEIGHT NATURALLY. Rodale Press, Emmaus, Pa. 1979.

This sensible and simple to follow book on weight loss draws on the newest developments in behavioral psychology, holistic health, and new-age nutrition. The reader learns how to use a variety of techniques to reinforce the effectiveness of this new eating program to lose weight naturally.

522. Broughton, Diane. CONFESSIONS OF A COMPULSIVE EATER. Elsevier-Nelson, New York. 1978.

This book is the outcome of taped conversations with a frenzied compulsive eater whose maniacal drive almost destroyed her and her family. The book demonstrates how society seems better able to deal with addictions to drugs, alcohol, and sex than to food addiction.

523. Bruch, Hilde. EATING DISORDERS: OBESITY, ANOREXIA NERVOSA, AND THE PERSON WITHIN. Basic Books, New York. 1979.

524. Collipp, Platon J., ed. CHILDHOOD OBESITY. 2nd ed. PSG Publications, Littleton, Mass. 1979.

525. Cooper, J. T., and Hagan, Paul. DR. COOPER'S FABULOUS FRUCTOSE DIET. M. Evans, New York. 1979.

The Fabulous Fructose Diet is meant as an aid in changing behavior that leads to overeating. The authors believe that difficulty in handling glucose is the weight watcher's nemesis.

526. Craddock, Denis. OBESITY AND ITS MANAGEMENT. 3rd ed. Churchill Livingstone, New York. 1978.

This book is an up-to-date and succinct summary of the etiology and management of both normal and refractory cases of obesity. General practitioners, hospital physicians, and dieticians will find this book extremely useful as a working manual during the day-to-day care of people with a weight problem.

527. Dolit, Alan. YOU CAN LOSE WEIGHT. Nellen Publishing, New York. 1979.

528. Ellis, C. Arthur, Jr., and Ellis, Leslie F. LOSE WEIGHT BY SURGERY. New ed. Heritage House, Tallahassee, Fla. 1977.

529. Foreyt, John P., ed. BEHAVIORAL TREATMENTS OF OBESITY: A PRACTICAL HANDBOOK. Pergamon, Elmsford, N.Y. 1977.

530. Gerrard, Don. ONE BOWL: A SIMPLE CONCEPT FOR CONTROL-LING BODY WEIGHT. Random House-Bookworks, New York. 1974.

This book presents a simple but unique method for controlling body weight based upon the common sensations of digestion. This concept helps to develop a new food attitude which will allow the loss of excess weight, satisfy food feeling and increase inner harmony.

531. Gilbert, Sara. FAT FREE: COMMON SENSE FOR YOUNG WEIGHT WORRIERS (Gr. 5, up). Macmillan, New York. 1978.

This book emphasizes the problems of dealing with over-weight adolescents and the difficulties in achieving weight control. Fat Free contains scientific information that helps explain what fat is and where it comes from and clarifies the relationship between the food eaten and the circumstances under which it was eaten.

532. Goldberg, Larry. GOLDBERG'S DIET CATALOG. Macmillan, New York. 1977.

533. Kraus, Barbara. CALORIES AND CARBOHYDRATES: A DICTIONARY OF 7500 BRAND NAMES AND BASIC FOODS WITH THEIR CALORIC AND CARBOHYDRATE COUNT. Rev. ed. New American Library, New York. 1979.

This useful compendium of over 7500 brand names and frequently eaten foods lists the caloric and carbohydrate counts of everything from Aquavit to Zwieback. Included are such brands as Sara Lee, McDonald's, and Duncan Hines.

534. Le Shan, Eda. WINNING THE LOSING BATTLE: WHY I WILL
     NEVER BE FAT AGAIN. T. Y. Crowell, New York. 1979.

     A leading family counselor provides a first-person ac-
     count of how she faced the terrors of being fat and of
     losing weight. She believes that fears and anxieties
     are the cause of overeating. Thus, the focus should be
     on the critical period before dieting. Emphasizing the
     importance of mental preparation for losing weight,
     Mrs. Le Shan claims that one must love the self beneath
     the veil of fat. This book offers the reader a day-to-
     day program of down-to-earth advice on how to become
     slim and how to remain that way.

535. Lindsey, Jan H., and Tear, June. FED UP WITH FAT.
     Revell, Old Tappan, N.J. 1978.

536. Rubin, Theodore I. ALIVE AND FAT AND THINNING IN
     AMERICA. Coward, McCann & Geoghegan, New York. 1978.

     This book describes the state of being a fat person in
     our culture today and provides the insights necessary
     to thinning--losing weight and sustaining weight loss.

537. Shedd, Charlie W. THE FAT IS IN YOUR HEAD. Word Books,
     Waco, Texas. 1977.

538. Stuelke, Richard G. THIN FOR LIFE. Baronet, New York.
     1977.

     The author introduces the reader to a new approach to
     weight loss called psychostructure--a system by which
     you gain control over the ingestion of food. The pro-
     gram encompasses a knowledge of calories, knowing how
     to react to food, how to determine how much and when
     to eat, where the pitfalls lie, and how to cope with
     them.

539. Stunkard, Albert J. I ALMOST FEEL THIN. Bull, Palo
     Alto, Calif. 1977.

540. Title, Stanley H., and Klein, Charles M. SENSIBLY·THIN.
Nelson-Hall, Chicago. 1979.

The practical premise of this book implies that given
the proper information, the reader can control his/her
weight.

541. Vassar, Charles C. HOW TO LOSE WEIGHT WHILE YOU SLEEP.
Pocket Books, New York. 1977.

542. Watson, Naomi. STOP DIETING! BEGIN LOSING WITH GOURMET
MAGIC. Butterfly Press, Houston, Texas. 1978.

543. Wolff, Jurgen M., and Lipe, Duane H. HELP FOR THE
OVERWEIGHT CHILD. Stein & Day, Briarcliff Manor, N.Y.
1978.

This workbook examines the causes and penalties of being
overweight. The author offers information about nutrition and exercise and about the psychology of weight
loss. Step-by-step instructions guide parents in good
eating and exercise habits to make slimmer, healthier,
and happier children.

Fasting

544. Anderson, Andy. FASTING CHANGED MY LIFE. Broadman Press, Nashville, Tenn. 1977.

545. Beall, James L. THE ADVENTURE OF FASTING. Revell, Old Tappan, N.J. 1974.

546. Cott, Allan; Agee, J.; and Boe, E. FASTING: A WAY OF LIFE. Bantam, New York. 1977.

547. Dobrzynski, Judith H. FASTING. Sovereign Books, New York. 1979.

This clear and simple guide to good nutrition reveals how fasting helps cure addictions to unnecessary food, revives our dulled senses, and guides us to sounder nutritional habits. One of the most appealing aspects of this book is the author's review of the history and religious uses of fasts.

548. Ehret, Arnold. INSTRUCTIONS FOR FASTING AND DIETING. Lust, Benedict, Greenwich, Conn. 1979.

549. Fulton, Alvenia M. THE FASTING PRIMER. 2nd ed. BCA Publications, Chicago. 1978.

550. Linn, Robert. THE LAST CHANCE DIET BOOK. Bantam, New York. 1977.

Why does one get fat and why does one stay fat? Dr. Linn answers these questions and offers a program for solving the problem. Diet fads and fallacies and the psychology of fasting are discussed. Who cannot fast, the dangers and history of fasting, and often-asked questions about fasting are included.

551. MacFadden, Bernarr. FASTING FOR HEALTH. Arc Books, New York. 1978.

"During my business activities in the last twenty-five years I cannot recall a single day's absence due to illness. This is all due to my ability to look ahead—to avoid disease by cleansing the body with fasting," so states the author of this intensely personal book.

The effects of fasting, when to and when not to fast, and how to break the fast are discussed intelligently.

552. Partee, Phillip E. THE LAYMAN'S GUIDE TO FASTING AND LOSING WEIGHT. Sprout Publications, Sarasota, Fla. 1979.

553. Ross, Shirley. FASTING. St. Martin's, New York. 1975.

Fasting is not a fad book, but a carefully researched examination of the fasting phenomenon. The author discusses in detail interviews with people who have fasted for as long as 57 days. The book outlines the proper procedures for fasting safely and explores every aspect of the subject from dieting to consciousness-raising.

554. Shelton, Herbert M. FASTING CAN SAVE YOUR LIFE. 2nd ed. Natural Hygiene Press, Chicago. 1978.

Every aspect of fasting is treated in this book, including reasons for fasting, where and when to fast, what to expect while fasting, and how to break a fast. Nine basic steps for fasting are spelled out and a section is included about whether or not children should fast.

555. Smith, J. Harold. FAST YOUR WAY TO HEALTH. Nelson, Thomas, Nashville, Tenn. 1979.

Vitamins

556. Benowicz, Robert J. VITAMINS AND YOU. Grosset & Dunlap, New York. 1978.

The author discusses the reasons why vitamins are essential to life and how vitamin requirements vary for each person's metabolism. The book reveals how methods of harvesting, processing, and preparing affect the vitamin content of food. The reader acquires a wealth of information about the subject and learns to choose between natural and synthetic vitamins.

557. Bock, Raymond F. VITAMIN E: KEY TO YOUTHFUL LONGEVITY. Arc Books, New York. 1977.

558. Cudipp, Edythe. VITAMINS. Grosset & Dunlap, New York. 1978.

559. DiCyan, Erwin. THE VITAMINS IN YOUR LIFE. Simon & Schuster, New York. 1975.

This recommended book is an invaluable survey of vitamins, minerals, toxicity levels, use of supplements and trace elements. The author, a drug consultant for over 30 years, writes conservatively yet is open-minded to alternative views such as those of Pauling, Hoffer, and others.

560. Elder, Susan B. VITAMIN C AND THEE. Dayton Labs, Dayton, Ohio. 1978.

561. Griffin, La Dean. PLEASE DR., I'D RATHER DO IT MYSELF WITH VITAMINS AND MINERALS. Hawkes Publishing, Salt Lake City, Utah. 1979.

562. Hunter, Carol. VITAMINS. Baronet, New York. 1977.

563. Lesser, Michael. NUTRITION AND VITAMIN THERAPY. Grove, New York. 1979.

This book on preventive medicine demonstrates the connection between poor nutritional habits and environmental pollutants to the resulting imbalances in the body. The author describes the vital components of body chemistry explaining each of the vitamins and minerals in layman's terms, and devotes special chapters to the role nutrition plays in allergies, blood sugar levels, mental and emotional disturbances, and sexual vitality.

564. Levy, Joseph V., and Bach-y-Rita, Paul. VITAMINS: THEIR USE AND ABUSE. Liveright, New York. 1976.

The authors, both biomedical professionals, attempt to answer all of the important questions about vitamins and to examine some common beliefs about their use. The aim is to equip readers with a critical attitude toward what vitamins do and do not do for them. The book provides descriptions of megavitamin therapy, vitamins and weight reduction, the common cold, aging, and mental illness. The reader will also find a table of recommended dietary allowances, a glossary of common terms, and a description of recent vitamin legislation.

565. Lilliston, Lynn. MEGAVITAMINS: A NEW KEY TO HEALTH. Fawcett, New York. 1976.

566. Mindell, Earl. EARL MINDELL'S VITAMIN BIBLE. Rawson Wade, New York. 1979.

567. Newbold, H. L. MEGA-NUTRIENTS FOR YOUR NERVES. McKay, New York. 1975.

568. Newbold, H. L. VITAMIN C AGAINST CANCER. Ballantine, New York. 1979.

This book offers evidence for the advantageous uses of Vitamin C. The author presents fascinating accounts of this vitamin therapy by leaders in the nutritional oncological field such as Linus Pauling, Albert Szent-Gyorgyi, and William Saccoman.

569. Passwater, Richard. SUPERNUTRITION: MEGAVITAMIN REVOLUTION. Pocket Books, New York. 1976.

570. Pauling, Linus. VITAMIN C, THE COMMON COLD AND THE FLU. W. H. Freeman, San Francisco. 1976.

This influential book, written by a Nobel prize-winning scientist, has changed the nutritional habits of

millions. In this book, direct and indirect evidence
is presented to support the conclusion that Vitamin C
protects the body. The general properties of the vitamin, how best to buy it, how to take it, and the attitude of the medical profession toward it are all
touched upon.

571. Prevention Magazine. THE COMPLETE BOOK OF VITAMINS.
     Rodale Press, Emmaus, Pa. 1980.

     This updated and enlarged encyclopedia of vitamin knowl-
     edge gives a complete description of each vitamin from
     its discovery to the latest therapeutic advances. The
     book provides information on how vitamins keep us
     healthy, how they react with other food elements, and
     describes numerous ailments treated successfully by
     vitamin therapy.

572. Shute, Wilfrid E., M.D. HEALTH PRESERVER, DEFINING THE
     VERSATILITY OF VITAMIN E. Rodale Press, Emmaus, Pa.
     1977.

     This book heralds the virtues of Vitamin E as an effec-
     tive treatment for a wide range of ailments. Readers
     will learn how Vitamin E prevents heart attacks, less-
     ens the side effects of diabetes, and halts the progress
     of gangrene in limbs devoid of circulation. Even astro-
     nauts have taken Vitamin E to minimize the undesirable
     effects of space flight.

573. Shute, Wilfrid E. YOUR CHILD AND VITAMIN E. Keats,
     New Canaan, Conn. 1979.

574. Takton, D. GREAT VITAMIN HOAX. Macmillan, New York.
     1967.

     The author conducted an economic and marketing study to
     determine the feasibility of successfully retailing
     vitamins. After extensive interviews with nutrition-
     ists, physicians, vitamin manufacturer's representa-
     tives, and government leaders, Mr. Takton unearthed
     incriminating evidence revealing the great vitamin
     hoax.

575. Timms, Moira, and Zar, Zachariah. NATURAL SOURCES:
     VITAMIN B-17/LAETRILE. Celestial Arts, Millbrae,
     Calif. 1978.

576. Wade, Carlson. FACT BOOK ON VITAMINS AND OTHER SUPPLE-
     MENTS. Keats, New Canaan, Conn. 1979.

     This book helps the reader understand the reasons food
     supplements can help create a healthier and longer life.

577. Wade, Carlson. VITAMIN E: THE REJUVENATION VITAMIN.
     Ace Books, New York. 1979.

578. Wintzler, Rich. THE VITAMIN BOOK. Simon & Schuster,
     New York. 1978.

HEALTH AREAS SPECIAL TO WOMEN

Biologically, women enjoy an exceptional position. They are stronger and live longer than men. Today, one woman in four outlives her eldest son. Projected for the year 2035 the population of older women will swell to 33.4 million, compared to a population of 22.4 million older men.

Women bear our children; they become the pivotal center for family unity and diligently groom future generations. Women are the largest consumers of health services, averaging 25 percent more visits to the doctor each year than men. Women take 50 percent more prescription drugs than men take and are admitted into hospitals more frequently.

Beyond being substantial consumers of health care, women make up 70 percent of all health workers and 75 percent of all hospital workers. Although more women work in the health industry, they do not occupy positions of power; for example, only 12 percent of the physicians in the U.S. are women.

Historically, childbearing and its attendant responsibilities have been the major occupation of most women. Even though childbirth is an event that happens thousands of times a day, it can have a profound and lasting effect on the health and well-being of women. In the past the medical profession directed the course of the pregnancy and determined the use of medication during delivery. Each phase of childbearing was handled by a different set of experts.

Today's women, exposed to new information and new attitudes, are exploring more natural courses of action for themselves and their children. Women are beginning to manage their nutritional requirement, medication intake, and other health needs with greater sophistication than ever before; and indeed the growing interest in natural childbirth has given rise to two alternative environments to the traditional hospital delivery room--the home and the hospital birthing room.

Self-help groups have been a significant source of
strength and learning for women who were formerly hesitant
to explore and experiment on their own. The self-help
movement has also sparked the development of women's
clinics. These clinics were formed by women for women and
evolved from a sense of frustration with the lack of personal health services.

The future will see a different set of economic and
social systems to support the increasing numbers of women
who will live and work longer. This shift in the lifestyle
of women will make inordinate demands on the health of
their bodies and minds, and it is to this need that particular attention should be focused on health areas special
to women.

HEALTH AREAS SPECIAL TO WOMEN

General

579. Anderson, Linda; Hjelm, Andrea; McGlone, Mary Ellen; Voyles, Bonnie; and Wilson, Linda. THE PERSON YOU ARE. PAR Inc., Providence, R.I. 1978.

This book offers advice to the woman seeking a career. The authors focus on the development of personal growth, the importance of self-presentation, and the complexities of interpersonal relations. The concluding section concentrates on learning how to integrate and use multiple skills.

580. Bermosk, Loretta Sue, and Porter, Sarah Ellen. WOMEN'S HEALTH AND HUMAN WHOLENESS. Appleton-Century-Crofts, New York. 1979.

The book presents effective methods for providing health care from birth to death, using procedures such as share-care, protocols, self-help, and other modalities from both Western and Eastern healing cultures.

The authors discuss the influence of sexism on women's health care and the development of women health professionals. This is an excellent book for those interested in the women's health movement.

581. Busby, Trent. BE GOOD TO YOUR BODY. Citadel Press, Secaucus, N.J. 1977.

This enlightening book on the mental and physical health of women discusses the multiple facets of female health and hygiene, especially as they pertain to sexuality. The author has spent 25 years as a practicing gynecologist.

582. DiMarco, Toni. THE CALIFORNIA WAY TO NATURAL BEAUTY.
Grosset & Dunlap, New York. 1976.

The author, an international fashion model and a student
of fine arts and architecture, demonstrates how to develop a "consciousness" of beauty. She feels that diets
and calorie-counting are counterproductive, and offers
personal advice about exercise and diet. Ms. DiMarco
provides a wealth of tips for mind and body.

583. Eckholm, Erik, and Newland, Kathleen. HEALTH: THE
FAMILY PLANNING FACTOR. (Worldwatch Institute Paper
#10.) Worldwatch Institute, Washington, D.C. 1977.

This excellent work is a product of Worldwatch Institute,
an independent, non-profit research organization created
to identify and focus attention on global problems. The
author discusses global perspectives of mothering, child-
birthing, abortion, and contraceptive safety.

584. Hunt, Vilma. WORK AND THE HEALTH OF WOMEN. CRC Press,
Boca Raton, Fla. 1979.

In this excellent book on health and the working woman,
the author discusses the demography of women workers;
ergonomics; physical, chemical, and biological environments; legal considerations bearing on health and em-
ployment of women workers; historical experience; and
future expectations.

585. MacKeith, Nancy, ed. THE NEW WOMEN'S HEALTH HANDBOOK.
Academy, Ltd., Chicago. 1978.

Written by women who are experts in their respective
fields, this book is considered a landmark in women's
self-help medicine. The editor provides knowledge and
essential medical information necessary to give women
the confidence to control their own bodies and their
lives.

Pregnancy and Childbirth

586. Arms, Suzanne. IMMACULATE DECEPTION. Houghton Mifflin Co., Burlington, Mass. 1975.

This excellent, comprehensive collection of essays on topics related to women and childbirth in America grew out of the author's need to understand and explain her own birth experience. The book is amply illustrated with photographs and the author quotes extensively from the experiences of individual women.

587. Ashdown-Sharp, Patricia. A GUIDE TO PREGNANCY AND PARENTHOOD FOR WOMEN ON THEIR OWN. Random House, New York. 1977.

588. Ballou, Judith. THE PSYCHOLOGY OF PREGNANCY. Lexington Books, Lexington, Mass. 1978.

589. Bing, Elizabeth. MOVING THROUGH PREGNANCY. Bantam, New York. 1976.

This book presents a series of useful exercises designed especially for the pregnant woman. The exercises, illustrated by photographs, have been developed by the author in her classes.

590. Bing, Elizabeth, and Colman, Libby. MAKING LOVE DURING PREGNANCY. Bantam, New York. 1977.

591. Bing, Elizabeth. SIX PRACTICAL LESSONS FOR AN EASIER CHILDBIRTH. Bantam, New York. 1977.

The author of this excellent instruction manual on childbirth was a pioneer in introducing the Lamaze method to America. The book is easy to follow, packed with information, and useful for review.

592. Birch, William G., and Meilach, Dona Z. DOCTOR DISCUSSES PREGNANCY. Budlong Press, Chicago. 1979.

593. Brennan, Barbara, and Heilman, Joan. COMPLETE BOOK OF MIDWIFERY. E. P. Dutton, New York. 1977.

The author describes her personal experiences in this book on midwifery. She discusses the role of midwives

and what a midwife can offer an expectant mother. This
well-illustrated book, written for the layperson, contains a listing of the addresses of nurse-midwifery
services in the U. S., plus a bibliography and index.

594. Brewer, Gail, and Brewer, Tom. WHAT EVERY PREGNANT
     WOMAN SHOULD KNOW: THE TRUTH ABOUT DIET AND DRUGS IN
     PREGNANCY. Penguin, New York. 1979.

595. Brewer, Gail S., ed. PREGNANCY AFTER THIRTY WORKBOOK.
     Rodale Press, Emmaus, Pa. 1978.

596. Brewster, Dorothy P. YOU CAN BREASTFEED YOUR BABY...
     EVEN IN SPECIAL SITUATIONS. Rodale Press, Emmaus, Pa.
     1979.

597. Cheetham, Juliet. UNWANTED PREGNANCY AND COUNSELLING.
     Routledge & Kegan, Boston. 1978.

598. Colman, Arthur, and Colman, Libby. PREGNANCY: THE
     PSYCHOLOGICAL EXPERIENCE. Bantam, New York. 1977.

     The Colmans describe the various stages of pregnancy,
     labor, and delivery, including the psychological compli-
     cations at each step. Separate chapters for mothers and
     for fathers are a unique feature of this book.

599. Davies, Margaret L., ed. MATERNITY: LETTERS FROM WORK-
     ING WOMEN. Norton, New York. 1979.

600. Dick-Read, Grantly. CHILDBIRTH WITHOUT FEAR. 4th ed.
     Harper & Row, New York. 1978.

     This book is considered a classic work on natural child-
     birth. The author describes the development of the
     child from conception to birth, the anatomy and physi-
     ology of mother and child during pregnancy and delivery,
     and the reasons for fear and painful labor when the
     mother is inadequately prepared for childbirth. The
     proper place of anaesthetics in natural childbirth is
     discussed.

601. Dilfer, Carol. YOUR BABY YOUR BODY. Crown, New York.
     1977.

602. Ebrahim, G. BREAST FEEDING: THE BIOLOGICAL OPTION.
     Schocken, New York. 1979.

603. Eiger, Marvin, and Olds, Sally. THE COMPLETE BOOK OF
     BREASTFEEDING. Bantam Books, New York. 1973.

     This book is a comprehensive examination of breast-
     feeding. The material is clearly written and the book
     includes photographs and a long bibliography.

604. Eloesser, Leo; Galt, Edith, and Hemingway, Isabel.
     PREGNANCY, CHILDBIRTH AND THE NEWBORN: A MANUAL FOR
     RURAL MIDWIVES. Inter-American Indian Institute,
     Mexico. 1973.

     This illustrated manual was originally developed to ac-
     company courses given in China to women with no more
     than a primary school education. The volume includes
     chapters on the anatomy and physiology of the female
     reproductive organs, the progress and conduct of preg-
     nancy and childbirth, and the care of the newborn.

605. Gazella, Jacqueline G. NUTRITION FOR THE CHILDBEARING
     YEAR. Woodland, Wayzata, Minn. 1979.

606. Gerrick, David J. PREGNANCY TESTING. Dayton Labs,
     Dayton, Ohio. 1978.

607. Gillespie, Clark. YOUR PREGNANCY MONTH BY MONTH.
     Harper & Row, New York. 1977.

608. Glas, Norbert. CONCEPTION, BIRTH AND EARLY CHILDHOOD.
     Anthroposophic Press, Inc., Spring Valley, N. Y. 1972.

     This book is a sensitive, intuitive account of the ef-
     fects the conception process has on the mother. The
     conceptual framework is based on Rudolf Steiner's
     Spiritual Science. The major part of the book is de-
     voted to the spiritual development of mother and child
     and an analysis of the newborn's developing his or her
     senses, will, and feeling.

609. Gots, Ronald E., and Gots, Barbara A. CARING FOR YOUR
     UNBORN CHILD. Bantam, New York. 1979.

610. Hambrick-Stowe, Elizabeth A. EXPECTING. Judson Press,
Valley Forge, Pa. 1979.

611. Hodson, Geoffrey. THE MIRACLE OF BIRTH. Theosophical
Publishing House, Wheaton, Ill. 1929.

The author, possibly one of the most intuitive, contemporary theosophists, presents his study of the
formation and development of the emotional, mental, and
physical aspects of a human being during the prenatal
period. The material is based on his observation of
one individual.

612. Howard, Marion. ONLY HUMAN: TEENAGE PREGNANCY AND
PARENTHOOD. Avon, New York. 1979.

613. Kahan, Stuart. THE EXPECTANT FATHER'S SURVIVAL KIT.
Sovereign Books, New York. 1979.

614. Kitzinger, Sheila. THE EXPERIENCE OF CHILDBIRTH.
Viking Penguin, New York. 1978.

This manual prepares the expectant mother for the physical and emotional aspects of childbirth. The author
describes the physiology of pregnancy, the development
of the fetus, and the successive stages of labor. Ms.
Kitzinger focuses on the psychological and marital ad-
justments of both wife and husband to parenthood and
the woman's changing relationship with her own mother.
The book contains a full discussion on the touch-
relaxation method, and the author adds many personal
accounts of labor recorded by pupils.

615. La Leche League. THE WOMANLY ART OF BREASTFEEDING.
La Leche League, Franklin Park, Ill. 1963.

The La Leche League, well-known in the natural childbirth movement, is the foremost exponent of breastfeeding. This manual was originally developed for mothers
too far away from a group to attend meetings and to
discuss the following topics: breastfeeding, planning
for the baby, nutrition for nursing mothers, common
worries and old wives' tales, the baby's arrival, the
mothering of the newborn, special circumstances, and the
father's role.

616. Lamaze, Ferdinand. PAINLESS CHILDBIRTH: THE LAMAZE
     METHOD. Contemporary Books, Chicago. 1970.

     Lamaze is the French physician who developed the most
     widely used method of natural childbirth. This book
     consists of a theoretical presentation of the physiology
     of childbirth along with transcriptions of the author's
     lectures. This is primarily a reference book.

617. Leboyer, Frederick. BIRTH WITHOUT VIOLENCE. Randam
     House, Westminster, Md. 1975.

     This important book directs the reader's attention to
     procedures being employed in hospitals all over the
     world. The author has developed revolutionary tech-
     niques for easing the birth trauma and shows exactly
     what can be done to replace the terror that has, until
     now, been taken for granted in the delivery of the new-
     born.

618. McCauley, Carole S. PREGNANCY AFTER THIRTY-FIVE.
     Pocket Books, New York. 1978.

619. MacIntyre, Sally. SINGLE AND PREGNANT: THE PREGNANCY
     CAREERS OF UNMARRIED WOMEN. Neale Watson, New York.
     1977.

620. Marzollo, Jean, ed. 9 MONTHS, 1 DAY, 1 YEAR. Harper &
     Row, New York. 1976.

     This book deals with the whole period of pregnancy,
     birth and that first special year as a new parent. The
     authors attempt to share feelings, facts, and opinions
     that invite the reader to react to and relate as part
     of their own experience. This book provides support,
     cheer, and companionship to both parents without the
     condescending and patronizing tone often found in
     doctors' books.

621. Mitchell, Ingrid. GIVING BIRTH TOGETHER: THE MODERN
     PARENTS' HOME PROGRAM OF NATURAL CHILDBIRTH EXERCISES.
     Seabury Press, New York. 1975.

     This manual on natural childbirth was written by one of
     the leaders in the European movement and complements the

currently available works on the Lamaze method. Six graded lessons are designed to aid the mother-to-be in developing the capacity to stay awake, aware, and in optimal control of her body during labor and childbirth. Photographs and line drawings illustrate the exercises and some of the physiology. Many case histories and a series of color photographs of an actual birth are included.

622. Nilsson, Lennart. A CHILD IS BORN. Delacorte, New York. 1975.

This collection of realistic photographs gives both an accurate and an artistic picture of the physical development of the fetus from conception to birth. Here, step-by-step, you can follow the stages of fetal development: formation of different organs, heartbeats, arm and leg movements, etc.

623. Price, Jane. YOU'RE NOT TOO OLD TO HAVE A BABY. Penguin, New York. 1978.

624. Rakowitz, Elly, and Rubin, Gloria S. LIVING WITH YOUR NEW BABY: A POSTPARTUM GUIDE FOR MOTHERS AND FATHERS. Watts Franklin, New York. 1978.

625. Raphael, Dana. THE TENDER GIFT: BREASTFEEDING. Schocken Books, New York. 1976.

The author devotes a great deal of this highly recommended volume to a comprehensive survey of past and present views on breastfeeding and breastfeeding from other cultures. Based on the author's research and experience, instructional material is offered on suggested nursing techniques.

626. Salmon, Margaret B. JOY OF BREASTFEEDING. Techkits, Demarest, N.J. 1979.

627. Shandler, Nina, and Shandler, Michael. YOGA FOR PREGNANCY AND BIRTH: A GUIDE FOR EXPECTANT PARENTS. Schocken Books, New York. 1979.

This excellent book for expectant parents is concerned with the presence of God within expectant mothers and

fathers and within their babies. The authors respon-
sibly delineate the systems and methods of yoga while
reminding the reader of the spirit of yoga.

628. Smith, David W. MOTHERING YOUR UNBORN BABY. Saunders,
Philadelphia. 1979.

629. Sousa, Marion. CHILDBIRTH AT HOME. Prentice-Hall,
Englewood Cliffs, N.J. 1976.

This is the most comprehensive, unified manual on child-
birth-at-home yet produced. The author provides practical information on preparations for the home birth.
The book provides prenatal nutrition and exercises,
along with descriptions of equipment and bedding. The
author tells how to recruit experienced medical super-
vision in the case of an emergency.

630. Stoppard, Miriam. DR. MIRIAM STOPPARD'S BOOK OF BABY
CARE. Atheneum, New York. 1977.

631. Thompson, Judi. HEALTHY PREGNANCY THE YOGA WAY.
Doubleday, New York. 1977.

The author, a mother of four children and a teacher of
yoga, presents a clear and thorough explanation of the
role yoga can play in maternal health. The importance
of relaxing, energizing during relaxation, meditating
and breathing correctly are emphasized. Basic rules
and warnings to expectant mothers are included; standing, sitting, and prone postures and exercises are
clearly illustrated in photographs of a pregnant model.

632. Whelan, Elizabeth M. THE PREGNANCY EXPERIENCE; THE
PSYCHOLOGY OF EXPECTANT PARENTHOOD. Norton, New York.
1978.

633. Williams, Phyllis S. NOURISHING YOUR UNBORN CHILD.
Nash Publishers, New York. 1974.

This book contains a wealth of information for every
mother or mother-to-be. It is a fact-filled, commonsense nutrition guide which covers the basic physiology
of childbearing, the management of pregnancy, childbirth, and the postpartum period. The author, a

registered nurse, explains the hazards and effects of
medications, illnesses, and infectious diseases and
provides a complete, in-depth discussion of foods with
the greatest nutritional value, plus information on
vitamin and mineral supplements.

HEALTH EDUCATION

If one waits long enough, the styles of yesteryear become the fashions of today. This phenomenon is happening now in the field of health education. The growing awareness of the value of self-help, prevention, and health promotion has fueled national interest in rediscovering health education. The profusion of available information allows individuals to recognize that they--not the experts-- have the option of making health-related decisions that can either heighten or diminish well-being.

The 1970s saw a decade of burgeoning public health-oriented bureaus and programs for health education. The government responded to the persistent public clamor for better health by creating public and private agencies devoted to furthering the thrust of health education. For example, in 1973, the President's Committee on Health Education advocated the establishment of a Bureau of Health Education within HEW and provided funds for a National Center for Health Education in the private sector.

At the same time in Europe, renewed interest in health education became an integral dimension of health policy and implementation. In 1974, "Operation Lifestyle" became Canada's ongoing public education campaign developed to encourage Canadians to preserve their health through improved lifestyle habits.

For thousands of years mankind has been concerned about preserving health. The present development has expanded traditional efforts in health education by introducing integrative phenomena. Today, a comprehensive integrative health education program still embraces topic information, i.e., diet, cleanliness, and disease control, but focuses on a combination of learning experiences to offer the individual and community options for adapting behavior for healthier lifestyles.

Health education, in the 20th century, means the selection of knowledge and the application of experience which will minimize risk, increase the potential for early intervention, and facilitate the effective use of the health care system for consumers.

141

HEALTH EDUCATION

General

634. Bauwens, Eleanor E., ed. THE ANTHROPOLOGY OF HEALTH.
C. V. Mosby, St. Louis, Mo. 1978.

The purpose of this volume is to educate and prepare
individuals who want to specialize in the field of medical anthropology. This excellently researched book
introduces behavioral science to the medical, nursing,
and other health professions, and contributes an important volume for the development of literature in medical
anthropology.

635. Brooks, Natalie, and Brooks, Stewart M. TURNER'S
PERSONAL AND COMMUNITY HEALTH. 15th ed. C. V. Mosby,
St. Louis, Mo. 1979.

636. Cornacchia, Harold J., and Staton, Wesley M. HEALTH
IN THE ELEMENTARY SCHOOLS. 5th ed. C. V. Mosby,
St. Louis, Mo. 1979.

This revised volume is designed to help meet present and
future demands for elementary classroom teachers and
supervisors. The book deals with the basic aspects of
school health education--curriculum, values, methods and
strategies, human and material resources, health services, and healthful school environment. New concepts
of health--holistic health and the addition of a spiritual dimension (values, moral issues, and humanism)
make this text stand apart from other books of its kind.

637. Dalis, Gus, and Strasser, Ben. TEACHING STRATEGIES FOR
VALUES AWARENESS AND DECISION MAKING IN HEALTH EDUCATION.
Charles B. Slack, Thorofare, N.J. 1977.

638. Engs, Ruth; Barnes, S. Eugene; and Wantz, Molly.
HEALTH GAMES STUDENTS PLAY: CREATIVE STRATEGIES FOR

143

HEALTH EDUCATION.   Kendall-Hunt, Dubuque, Iowa.
1976.

This imaginative publication is primarily aimed at the
practicing or student health educator teaching grades
6 through 12. It contains a variety of structured experiences, simulation games, and experiential exercises.
These techniques are geared to the secondary school
level but, by adjusting content or terminology, can be
readily adapted to elementary or college levels. The
text provides examples of the types of exercises which
can help stimulate the teacher of health education to
create an assortment of interesting and meaningful activities for students.

639. Ford, Beryl I. HEALTH EDUCATION: A SOURCE BOOK FOR
     TEACHING. Pergamon, Elmsford, N.Y. 1978.

640. Galli, Nicholas. FOUNDATIONS AND PRINCIPLES OF HEALTH
     EDUCATION. Wiley, New York. 1978.

This book is a basic reference for those who are preparing for a career in health education and is an excellent
resource for the general reader interested in the field.
Discussion ranges from health and disease to legal
foundations and opportunities in health education.

641. Gay, John; Wantz, Molly; Slobol, Harold; and Hooper,
     Carol. CURRENT HEALTH PROBLEMS. Saunders,
     Philadelphia. 1979.

The basic premise of this text suggests that health
education, in addition to the presentation of basic
cognitive and affective information, should go one step
further by assisting students in developing decision-
making skills. The text offers the student a basic
understanding of the meaning of health and its application to the world, the nation, and the individual. The
author examines the many modes used in the solution of
a health problem and then establishes a specific model
for solving health-related problems.

642. Green, Lawrence W.; Kreuter, Marshall W.; Reeds,
     Sigrid G.; and Partridge, Kay B. HEALTH EDUCATION

PLANNING. Mayfield Publishing, Palo Alto, Calif.
1979.

The authors define health education activities as a
combination of learning experiences designed to make
people voluntarily adapt behavior conducive to health
and well-being. Guidelines are developed to help the
reader understand how planners design and organize
health education activities. This book explains why
the process of health education involves more than mere
information dissemination.

643. Hamburg, Joseph, ed. REVIEW OF ALLIED HEALTH EDUCATION:
2. University of Kentucky Press, Lexington, Ky. 1977.

This second book in a series is designed to provide a
current appraisal of the developments in allied health
education and research, through original articles contributed by recognized leaders in the field. This review seeks, by means of enlightened commentary, to help
bind the health professions into a true alliance.

644. Henkel, Barbara O.; Means, Richard K.; Sawrey, James M.;
and Smolinsky, Jack. FOUNDATIONS OF HEALTH SCIENCE.
3rd ed. Allyn & Bacon, New York. 1977.

This text will help the reader to evaluate the concept
of prevention and to practice preventive behavior. This
third edition is a valuable adjunct to the college instructor in his effort to increase levels of health
knowledge, create attitudes favorable to desirable
health practices and to motivate young adults to improve
their health behavior.

645. Insel, Paul, and Roth, Walton T. HEALTH IN A CHANGING
SOCIETY. Mayfield Publ., Palo Alto, Calif. 1976.

646. Insel, Paul M., and Roth, Walton T. CORE CONCEPTS IN
HEALTH. 2nd ed. Mayfield Publ., Palo Alto, Calif.
1979.

647. Jones, Kenneth L.; Shainberg, Louis W.; and Byer,
Curtis O. PRINCIPLES OF HEALTH SCIENCE. Harper & Row,
New York. 1975.

Designed for the classroom, this text provides detailed
instructional objectives at the beginning of each chapter and complete outlines of all chapters are presented
as summaries. Pronunciation, derivations, and meanings
of important terms are given in the end-of-chapter
glossaries.

648. Jones, Kenneth L. DIMENSIONS: A CHANGING CONCEPT OF
HEALTH. 4th ed. Harper & Row, New York. 1979.

This book, intended for college health courses, provides
a broad background and stimulus for enlightened classroom discussion. The author shows a decided shift in
education away from the anatomical and physiological
and toward the behavioral and sociological aspects of
health.

649. Kime; Schlaadt, Richard G.; and Tritsch, Leonard G.
HEALTH INSTRUCTION: AN ACTION APPROACH. Prentice-Hall,
Englewood Cliffs, N.J. 1977.

650. Lazes, Peter, ed. THE HANDBOOK OF HEALTH EDUCATION.
Aspen Systems, Germantown, Md. 1979.

651. Lunin, Lois F., ed. HEALTH SCIENCES AND SERVICES: A
GUIDE TO INFORMATION SOURCES. Gale Research, Detroit.
1979.

This book is an organized inventory of available information resources, publications, data bases, and organizations in the health sciences and services. Such resources can be used to obtain information for research,
education, patient care, administration, and planning.

652. McGrath, Ruth E. DEVELOPING CONCEPTS OF HEALTH IN EARLY
CHILDHOOD. DOK Publishing, Buffalo, N.Y. 1977.

653. Phillips, David S. BASIC STATISTICS FOR HEALTH SCIENCE
STUDENTS. W. H. Freeman, San Francisco. 1978.

654. Rash, J. Keogh, and Pigg, R. Morgan. HEALTH EDUCATION
CURRICULUM: A GUIDE FOR CURRICULUM DEVELOPMENT IN HEALTH
EDUCATION. Wiley, New York. 1979.

This book provides guidelines for the health educator

who is concerned with developing the health education
curriculum.

655. Read, Donald; Simon, Sidney B.; and Goodman, Joel B.
HEALTH EDUCATION: THE SEARCH FOR VALUE. Prentice-Hall,
Englewood Cliffs, N.J. 1977.

656. Read, Donald, and Simon, Sidney B. HUMANISTIC EDUCATION
SOURCEBOOK. Prentice-Hall, Englewood Cliffs, N.J. 1975.

For the first time in one volume the authors present a
combination of the most innovative thinking and research on the humanistic approach to education. Read
and Simon provide an invaluable summation of the work
done to date, its current influence, and its implications for our educational future.

657. Read, Donald A., and Greene, Walter H. CREATIVE
TEACHING IN HEALTH. 2nd ed. Macmillan, New York. 1975.

This book focuses on the role and responsibility of the
classroom teacher as a major force in the creative
teaching-learning environment. The authors include a
good deal of background information on crucial health
problems and provide curriculum recommendations in the
form of priority concepts.

658. READINGS IN HEALTH, 80 - 81. Annual Editions. Dushkin
Publishing, Guilford, Conn. 1980.

Readings in Health, 80 - 81 is one in a series of
over 25 volumes, each providing convenient, inexpensive
access to a wide range of carefully selected articles
from some of the most important magazines, newspapers,
and journals published today. Fifty-nine interesting,
well-illustrated articles written by knowledgeable
scientists, health educators, researchers, and writers
provide effective and useful perspectives on the important health issues of the day.

659. Rosenkrantz, Barbara G., ed. SELECTIONS FROM THE HEALTH
EDUCATION SERIES: AN ORIGINAL ANTHOLOGY. Arno, New
York. 1977.

660. Scott, Gwendolyn D., and Carlo, Mona W. LEARNING -
     FEELING - DOING: DESIGNING CREATIVE LEARNING EXPERIENCES
     FOR ELEMENTARY HEALTH EDUCATION. Prentice-Hall, Engle-
     wood Cliffs, N.J. 1978.

661. Scott, Gwendolyn D., and Carlo, Mona W. ON BECOMING A
     HEALTH EDUCATOR. 2nd ed. Wm. C. Brown, Dubuque, Iowa.
     1979.

     It is the intent of the authors to nudge the reader to
     look beyond the bonds of traditional educational experi-
     ences and to consider embracing a philosophy of change,
     with emphasis on student involvement in learning and
     evaluation. This book is an excellent stimulant and
     support for those involved in school or community health
     education.

662. Sorochan, Walter D., and Bender, Stephen J. TEACHING
     ELEMENTARY HEALTH SCIENCE. 2nd ed. Addison-Wesley,
     Reading, Mass. 1979.

     This second edition places new emphasis on the specific
     areas of preparation deemed essential to the development
     of a competent elementary health educator. The authors
     have carefully structured the material so that even the
     most uninformed will be aware that a great deal can be
     done to assist children in attaining optimal well-being.
     The text is divided into five parts: 1) the meaning of
     health, 2) elementary child, 3) physical development,
     4) emotional-social development, and 5) development of
     values.

663. WHO 27th World Health Assembly, 1974. PROMOTING HEALTH
     IN THE HUMAN ENVIRONMENT: TECHNICAL DISCUSSIONS REVIEW.
     (Edited by Evang, Karl, and Meyer, Evelyn E.) World
     Health, Albany, N.Y. 1975.

HEALTH AND THE ENVIRONMENT

The threat of toxic factors in the environment is
ubiquitous. During a lifetime people are exposed to many
formidable health risks. Edward I of England in 1306
issued a proclamation banning the burning of "sea-coales"
(chunks of coal found along the seashore) because of their
health hazards. John Evelyn in 1661 attributed a shortened
life expectancy to smoke pollution. Erik Eckholm put into
perspective the correlation of environment to health when
he wrote, "Indeed in creating its way of life, each society
creates its way of death."

Without environmental access to adequate food or safe
water supplies, many illnesses and dysfunctions would deci-
mate a population; inadequate sanitation systems would
spread pestilence and disease. Industrial wastes that
cause air and water pollution, and manufacturing processes
that produce potentially harmful substances constantly
threaten to undermine health and well-being.

Environmentalists estimate that adequate public protection would lessen by as much as 20 percent all premature
deaths and significantly reduce the incidence of disease
and disability. Improvements in sanitation, housing,
water, and food production have been compromised by rapid
industrial and technological development. Accelerated
social changes, increased population, and intensification
of urban population have created many new challenges to
health. Oddly enough, the present danger from an accumulation of toxic substances in water and food supplies is
the long lag time (20 years or more) in the manifestation
of damage to a population. Years of exposure to such
phenomena are surreptitiously undermining the health and
well-being of society.

Eighty percent of Americans who live in urban environments coexist with gases and matter polluting the air and
water. Those industrial giants which provide society with
a means to modern living are the same providers of the
toxic wastes which discharge into our rivers and pollute
our air.

149

Probably the most widely discussed effect of hazardous substances is cancer. As the late John Knowles pointed
out, over 80 percent of human cancers are caused either
directly or indirectly by environmental factors. To
Knowles, "environmental factors" include cancer-provoking
substances in the foods and drugs we consume, the air we
breathe, the water we drink, the occupations we pursue,
and the habits we follow.

HEALTH AND THE ENVIRONMENT

General

664. Altman, Irwin, and Wohlwill, Joachim F., eds. HUMAN
BEHAVIOR AND ENVIRONMENTS: ADVANCES IN THEORY AND
RESEARCH. Plenum, New York. 1976.

This first book of a series presents information from
diverse sources on environmental and behavioral topics
and makes this knowledge accessible in a single publication to researchers and professionals. This volume
covers topics such as environmental attitudes and environmental aesthetics; perceptual aspects of land use;
environmental change and the aged; ecological psychology applied to institutional settings, recreation, and
work environment.

665. Baker, P. T., ed. MAN IN THE ANDES: A MULTIDISCIPLINARY
STUDY OF HIGH-ALTITUDE QUECHUA. Academy Press,
Chatsworth, Calif. 1976.

The material in this volume consists of contributions
from 17 scientists who participated in a multidisciplinary study of the biology of human populations at high
altitudes in southern Peru.

666. Berry, James; Osgood, David W.; and St. John, Philip A.
CHEMICAL VILLAINS: A BIOLOGY OF POLLUTION. C. V. Mosby,
St. Louis, Mo. 1974.

667. Calabrese, Edward J. METHODOLOGICAL APPROACHES TO
DERIVING ENVIRONMENTAL AND OCCUPATIONAL HEALTH STAND-
ARDS. Wiley, New York. 1978.

This book deals with the biomedical basis for environmental standards. The text includes a model for standard setting for both environmental and occupational
pollutants, provides a discussion of the concept of
high-risk groups, offers an assessment of the extent to
which chemical interactions occur in the air and focuses

151

on toxicological issues, drinking water standards, and
research by the National Institute for Occupational
Safety and Health (NIOSH) and other agencies.

668. Cannon, Helen, and Hopps, Howard C., eds. GEOCHEMICAL
ENVIRONMENT IN RELATION TO HEALTH AND DISEASE. Geologi-
cal Society of America, Boulder, Colo. 1972.

669. Eckholm, Erik P. THE PICTURE OF HEALTH: ENVIRONMENTAL
SOURCES OF DISEASE. Norton, New York. 1977.

Sponsored by the United Nations Environmental Program,
this book maintains that health is influenced less by
MD's and drugs than by our social and physical environment. Sample topics are undernutrition, poor sanitation,
the unnatural history of tobacco, cancer, and family
planning.

670. Fitzpatrick, Malcolm S. ENVIRONMENTAL HEALTH PLANNING:
COMMUNITY DEVELOPMENT BASED ON ENVIRONMENTAL AND HEALTH
PRECEPTS. Ballinger, Cambridge, Mass. 1978.

This book describes a plan for long range solutions to
environmental problems. The author gives the reader an
understanding of the systematic, hierarchial process by
which material on environment and health must be gath-
ered, analyzed, and applied in order to use our scarce
resources wisely in the near future.

671. Hinkle, L. E., and Loring, W. C. EFFECTS OF MAN-MADE
ENVIRONMENT ON HEALTH AND BEHAVIOR. International
Ideas, Philadelphia. 1979.

This book is the result of attempts by the Public Health
Service (PHS) to identify factors that relate to health
and disease or to safety and injury found in neighbor-
hoods of urban residents. An objective of the undertak-
ing was to include planned change or preventive intervention in guidelines for planners, architects, developers, social workers, and residents.

672. Luft, Harold S. POVERTY AND HEALTH: ECONOMIC CAUSES AND
CONSEQUENCES OF HEALTH PROBLEMS. Ballinger, Cambridge,
Mass. 1978.

673. McGee, Charles T. HOW TO SURVIVE MODERN TECHNOLOGY.
     Ecology Press, Alamo, Calif. 1979.

674. Moser, Leo J. THE TECHNOLOGY TRAP. Nelson-Hall,
     Chicago. 1979.

     This book makes a plea for human accountability in en-
     vironmental studies. The author believes that these
     studies should consider patterns of thought and tech-
     nological processes; psychological needs and methods of
     analysis; chemical tolerances and industrial costs.
     The author clearly shows the relation between mind and
     environment, demonstrating how the human mind has af-
     fected the environment and how challenges of past en-
     vironments shaped the contours of the human mind.

675. National Research Council, Division of Medical Sciences.
     OZONE AND OTHER PHOTOCHEMICAL OXIDANTS. (Series:
     Medical and Biological Effects of Environmental Pollut-
     ants.) National Academy of Sciences, Washington, D.C.
     1977.

676. Schroeder, Henry A. THE POISONS AROUND US: TOXIC METALS
     IN FOOD, AIR AND WATER. Keats, New Canaan, Conn.
     1978.

     This book is concerned primarily with the effects of
     pollutants on human health and is based on a knowledge
     of metals and their toxicity (especially the use of low-
     level doses of metals given for a lifetime).

677. Shakman, Robert. WHERE YOU LIVE MAY BE HAZARDOUS TO
     YOUR HEALTH. Stein & Day, Briarcliff Manor, N.Y. 1978.

678. Trieff, Norman M., ed. ENVIRONMENT AND HEALTH. Ann
     Arbor Science, Ann Arbor, Mich. 1980

679. Waldbott, George L. HEALTH EFFECTS OF ENVIRONMENTAL
     POLLUTANTS. 2nd ed. C. V. Mosby, St. Louis, Mo. 1978.

     This book on environmental pollutants should be of in-
     terest to safety personnel in government and industry
     as well as to attorneys involved with pollution problems.
     The new edition, valuable to physicians and students of

environmental health, includes information on noise
pollution, new data on dioxins, aflatoxins, and micro-
wave radiation.

680. WHO Expert Committee, Geneva, 1973. HEALTH ASPECTS OF
ENVIRONMENTAL POLLUTION CONTROL--PLANNING AND IMPLEMENT-
ATION OF NATIONAL PROGRAMMES: REPORT. World Health,
Albany, N.Y. 1974.

681. WHO Study Group, Geneva, 1974. EARLY DETECTION OF
HEALTH IMPAIRMENT IN OCCUPATIONAL EXPOSURE TO HEALTH
HAZARDS: REPORT. World Health, Albany, N.Y. 1975.

682. WHO Study Group, Geneva, 1974. HEALTH HAZARDS FROM NEW
ENVIRONMENTAL POLLUTANTS: REPORT. World Health, Albany,
N.Y. 1976.

683. Witters, Weldon L., and Jones-Witters, Patricia.
ENVIRONMENTAL BIOLOGY: THE HUMAN FACTOR. 2nd ed.
Kendall-Hunt, Dubuque, Iowa. 1978.

This book which evolved from a course on Human Biology
at Ohio University includes such topics as communities,
niches, ecosystems, food chains, food webs, recycling
in nature, biomes, and ecological succession. The
authors believe that population and attitude are the two
major reasons the ecosystems of the world are in danger
today.

HEALTH IN INDUSTRY

The workplace, once the essential means to a liveli-
hood, has evolved to fill other important needs in the
lives of the worker: status, self-respect, and mental and
physical well-being. The physical and mental health of
the worker has assumed a proportion of interest even greater
than wages.

Many of the almost 100 million workers in the United
States are exposed to a variety of occupational health
risks. Some workers are exposed to carcinogenic agents or
circumstances that can produce pulmonary or other diseases;
others work in settings that generate adverse psychological
effects such as noise, crowding, boredom, stress- or job-
related pressure.

Each year 100,000 Americans die because of illness
associated with work, and another 400,000 develop new cases
of occupational illnesses. Because the link between illness and work often goes unrecognized, these figures may
be only the tip of the proverbial iceburg.

Accident and injury also take their toll. About 13,000
American workers die annually from work-related injuries
and another nine million are seriously affected by accidents
that require medical care or result in loss of work.

The installation of mechanical and technical devices
can control some occupational hazards, accidents and injuries, but effective prevention strategies require the
concerted efforts of employers, employees, unions, and
regulatory bodies. Moreover, many organizations and
agencies are recognizing the value of health promotion
measures and are taking steps to provide worksite programs.
Programs that consist of health education techniques offer
opportunities for physical fitness and provide screening
tests for hypertension, cholesterol, and heart disease.
Other programs focus attention on weight loss and the control of drinking and smoking.

Many enlightened employers are concerned with the
inability of employees to handle inordinate amounts of

155

stress in and out of the workplace and offer workers training in meditation, relaxation techniques, and coping mechanisms. Some programs offer the services of psychiatrists
and psychologists to help employees better handle the
pressures of work.

Perhaps one of the most promising developments that
has contributed to well-being at the workplace is the
evolution of worker participation in the decision-making
process. The workplace is a natural schoolroom for the
implementation of health education options because social
values and behaviors are delineated by the group with whom
we spend most of our waking and working day.

HEALTH IN INDUSTRY

General

684. Anton, Thomas. OCCUPATIONAL SAFETY AND HEALTH
MANAGEMENT. McGraw-Hill, New York. 1979.

685. Ashford, Nicholas A. CRISIS IN THE WORKPLACE:
OCCUPATIONAL DISEASE AND INJURY. MIT Press, Cambridge,
Mass. 1976.

This book actually incorporates four reports reflecting
four points of view that occupational-health-and-safety
decisionmakers might take depending on their back-
grounds. Fortunately for the reader, a summary followed by a helpful introduction is provided.

The book deals in turn with the economic, legal, and
political aspects of the implementations of the
Occupational Safety and Health Act of 1970; examines
the problems of manpower development; and describes some
of the important activities of the private sectors.
Special sections discuss the foreign experience and
special problems of agricultural workers.

686. Beyer, Janice M., and Trice, Harrison M. IMPLEMENTING
CHANGE: ALCOHOLISM POLICIES IN WORK ORGANIZATIONS. Free
Press, New York. 1978.

This book reports on a study of a legislative effort
designed to implement change on the issue of alcoholism
in the workplace. The research focuses on deliberate
and planned change rather than spontaneous change. The
authors discuss the change process, sampling, data collection, statistics, stages of implementation, roles of
directions, and interorganizational relations.

687. Brisolara, Ashton. THE ALCOHOLIC EMPLOYEE: A HANDBOOK OF
HELPFUL GUIDELINES. Human Science Press, New York. 1978.

This handbook is for people interested in the relief and

157

prevention of human problems and economic losses in
industry due to alcoholism. It describes the ramifica-
tions of the problem, presents an overall picture of
excessive drinking in industry, and offers some possible solutions. The author has studied the problem
carefully and prescribes in concise form a method of
approaching the occupational alcoholism problem with a
view toward saving industry billions of dollars.

688. Collis, Edgar L., and Greenwood, Major. THE HEALTH OF
     THE INDUSTRIAL WORKER. Arno, New York. 1977.

689. De Reamer, Russell. MODERN SAFETY AND HEALTH TECH-
     NOLOGY. Wiley, New York. 1979.

690. Peterson, Jack E. INDUSTRIAL HEALTH. Prentice-Hall,
     Englewood Cliffs, N.J. 1977.

691. Plant, Martin A. DRINKING CAREERS: OCCUPATIONS,
     DRINKING HABITS AND DRINKING PROBLEMS. Methuen, New
     York. 1979.

     The author is concerned with the relationship between
     an individual's drinking habits and social setting.
     The information in this book is empirical rather than
     theoretical.

692. Schramm, Carl J.; Mandell, Wallace; and Archer, Janet.
     WORKERS WHO DRINK. Lexington Books, Lexington, Mass.
     1978.

     This volume reports the results of a demonstration and
     research project undertaken to 1) explore a new concept
     in the organization of alcoholism treatment services,
     and 2) develop basic data on the labor force behavior
     of alcoholic workers.

693. Shostak, Arthur B. BLUE-COLLAR STRESS. Addison-
     Wesley, Reading, Mass. 1979.

     The author explores the current impact of major stress-
     ors on the working lives of white, blue-collar, American
     men. The book identifies objective and subjective
     stressors in work (compensation inadequacy, health and
     safety hazards, etc.) and discusses labor's role both as

a source and antidote to stress. Chapters analyze
physical and mental health issues, as well as stressors
created by new ecological and environmental controversies and spotlights several ongoing or prospective reforms likely to help workers lead less stressful lives.

694. Smith, Robert S. THE OCCUPATIONAL SAFETY AND HEALTH
ACT: ITS GOALS AND ITS ACHIEVEMENTS. American Enter-
prise Institute for Public Policy Research, Washington,
D.C. 1976.

695. Trice, Harrison M., and Roman, Paul M. SPIRIT AND
DEMONS AT WORK: ALCOHOL AND OTHER DRUGS ON THE JOB.
2nd ed. Cornell University, New York School of Industrial Relations, Ithaca, N.Y. 1979.

The authors present a comprehensive review of the impact
of alcohol and drugs in the workplace. This volume provides solid, practical guidance for intervening with
employees whose work performance is impaired by either
alcohol or drug abuse. Executives, managers, and supervisors, as well as counselors of troubled employees will
find this book very useful, especially the chapter outlining the technique of "constructive confrontation."

696. Warshaw, Leon J. MANAGING STRESS. Addison-Wesley,
Reading, Mass. 1979.

The book is intended to help managers on all levels
to recognize, appreciate, and control stress situations
in the workplace. The author suggests various kinds of
programs to ameliorate the effects of stress. Managers
are able to perform their roles more effectively by
examining the sources and effects of stress on the
organization and its personnel.

Mental Health in Industry

697. Carone, Pasquale, ed. THE EMOTIONALLY TROUBLED
EMPLOYEE: A CHALLENGE TO INDUSTRY. State University
of New York Press, Albany, N.Y. 1976.

698. Follman, Joseph F. HELPING THE TROUBLED EMPLOYEE.
American Management, New York. 1979.

This book discusses how to identify the troubled employee and examines the significant role that employers and
labor unions can play in helping. It describes various
types of mental disorders, their causes, and prevention.
The author looks at the incidence and economic costs of
people with mental disorders, the types of treatment
available, where to go for help, and how to finance
mental health care.

699. Frew, David R. MANAGEMENT OF STRESS: USING TM AT WORK.
Nelson-Hall, Chicago. 1977.

700. Kornhauser, Arthur. MENTAL HEALTH OF THE INDUSTRIAL
WORKER: A DETROIT STUDY. Krieger, Huntington, N.Y.
1965.

This book is concerned with the psychological condition
of workers in modern mass-production industry. The
author attempts to assess and compare the mental health
of men at higher and lower skill levels, with special
attention to the human effects of routine production
jobs.

The book is addressed not only to social scientists
interested in the human problems of industry but equally
to all thoughtful citizens concerned with wise social
policy affecting the welfare of working people. The
inherent frustrations of our great technology result
from unchallenging routine jobs and passive goalless
occupations.

701. Landy, Frank, and Trumbo, Don. A PSYCHOLOGY OF WORK
BEHAVIOR. Dorsey Press, Homewood, Ill. 1976.

702. Levinson, Harry. EMOTIONAL HEALTH: IN THE WORLD OF
WORK. Harper & Row, New York. 1964.

703. Levinson, Harry; Price, Charlton; Munden, Kenneth;
     Mandl, Harold; and Solley, Charles. MAN, MANAGEMENT AND
     MENTAL HEALTH. Harvard University Press, Cambridge,
     Mass. 1962.

     This classic study explores, describes, and interprets
     some of the experiences that affect the mental health
     of people at work in one industrial organization. The
     authors see mental health as being primarily related to
     a person's self image and his feelings about the world
     around him and his place in it; about his experiences
     while earning a living for himself and his dependents.
     This study guides the reader in an understanding of the
     psychological relationship of a person to the organiza-
     tion in which he works. The authors suggest ways in
     which management can contribute to mental health.

704. Lofquist, Lloyd H., and David, Rene V. ADJUSTMENT TO
     WORK: A PSYCHOLOGICAL VIEW OF MAN'S PROBLEMS IN A WORK-
     ORIENTED SOCIETY. Irvington, New York. 1979.

705. Mayo, Elton. THE SOCIAL PROBLEMS OF AN INDUSTRIAL
     CIVILIZATION. Arno, New York. 1977.

     In this classic volume, the author explores some of the
     complexities of human relationships in industry and
     society.

706. McLean, Alan A. WORK STRESS. Addison-Wesley Series
     Publishing Co., Reading, Mass. 1979.

     The author translates medical-psychiatric data on job-
     related stress into understandable, useful information
     for the general public. The book identifies the major
     variables of job stress and suggests methods of assess-
     ing stressors, handling stress reactions, and averting
     stress reactions before they occur. It also contains
     checklists which readers can use to determine how much
     work stress they face every day.

707. Neff, Walter S. WORK AND HUMAN BEHAVIOR. 2nd ed.
     Aldine Publ., Chicago. 1979.

708. Noland, Robert L. INDUSTRIAL MENTAL HEALTH AND EMPLOYEE
     COUNSELLING. Human Science Press, New York. 1973.

709. Norfolk, Donald. STRESS FACTOR. Simon & Schuster,
     New York. 1979.

710. Oates, Wayne E. CONFESSIONS OF A WORKAHOLIC.
     Abingdon, Nashville, Tenn. 1978.

     This book discusses the workaholic, wives and family
     lives of workaholics, and the threatening weekends.
     The author attempts to offer suggestions for remaking
     the life of the workaholic.

711. Oates, Wayne E. WORKAHOLICS: MAKE LAZINESS WORK FOR
     YOU. Doubleday, New York. 1978.

     An excellent book to read for those who feel shackled
     to their work. The author creatively discusses lazi-
     ness, vacations, free time, and "goofing off" in all
     good conscience.

712. O'Toole, James, ed. WORK: THE QUALITY OF LIFE.
     MIT Press, Cambridge, Mass. 1974.

     The consensus in this compilation of papers, based
     on Work in America, a report published by an HEW task
     force, reveals that the organization of work is ad-
     versely affecting the mental and physical health,
     family stability, and political behavior of many Amer-
     icans. The papers discuss problems of dissatisfied
     American workers, work and health, redesign of job,
     education and work, and federal work strategies.

713. Rusch, Frank R., and Mithaug, Dennis E. VOCATIONAL
     TRAINING FOR MENTALLY RETARDED ADULTS: A BEHAVIOR
     ANALYTIC APPROACH. Research Press, Champaign, Ill.
     1979.

714. Shostak, Arthur B. BLUE COLLAR STRESS. Addison-
     Wesley, Reading, Mass. 1979.

     The author explores the current impact of major stress-
     ors in the working lives of white, blue-collar American
     men. The book identifies objective and subjective
     stressors in work (compensation inadequacy, health
     and safety hazards, etc.) and discusses labor's role
     both as a source and antidote to stress. Chapters

analyze physical and mental health issues, as well as stressors created by new ecological and environmental controversies, and spotlights several ongoing or prospective reforms likely to help workers lead less stressful lives.

715. Simonson, Ernst, and Weiser, Philip C. PSYCHOLOGICAL ASPECTS AND PHYSIOLOGICAL CORRELATES OF WORK AND FATIGUE. Charles C Thomas, Springfield, Ill. 1976.

716. Stein, Leon, ed. WORK, ITS REWARDS AND DISCONTENTS. Arno, New York. 1977.

717. Warr, Peter, and Walls, Toby. WORK AND WELL-BEING. Penguin, New York. 1976.

The authors write about the quality of working life through an examination of work satisfaction and mental health of individual employees. Research investigations provide information about possible ways of satisfying both the workers' aspirations and the needs of the organization which employs them.

718. Wilson, Howard. COUNSELING EMPLOYEES. Administrative Research Associates, Irvine, Calif. 1973.

719. Zaetz, Jay L. OCCUPATIONAL ACTIVITIES TRAINING MANUAL: FOR SEVERELY RETARDED ADULTS. Charles C Thomas, Springfield, Ill. 1969.

ILLNESS AND DISEASE PREVENTION

Prevention is an idea whose time has come.

Within the practical grasp of most Americans are a
few simple measures to enhance the prospects of their
health and well-being such as the following practices:

- Moderate dietary changes to reduce intake of fat,
  sugar, salt, and calories
- Moderate exercise
- Elimination of smoking
- Moderate use of alcohol

Practices to prevent illness and promote health have
been recorded in ancient Chinese texts, and followers of
the healing arts have flourished in classical Greece. For
example, 4,000 years ago, the Yellow Emperor of China
chose to support practices and systems that nourished the
well rather than to support techniques that treated the
sick.

The sanitary reforms of the last half of the 19th
century, and the use of vaccines in the 20th century are
examples of advances in prevention. Following World War
II, interest in prevention waned because the chronic illnesses that have predominated our "sick lists" did not lend
themselves to simple causes or solutions.

In 1900, of the 10 major causes of death, six were
either infectious or related to infectious processes. In
1970, none of the 10 major causes of death was infectious:
heart disease, cancer, and accidents swell the list; while
yesterday's scourges, such as smallpox, diptheria, and
polio are no longer a threat.

Many, but not all, health risks are within the control
of the individual. However, the socio-economic, genetic,
and environmental risks that can contribute to illness are
beyond control. Cancer, for example, is surely the illness
most feared by Americans. One in four will develop cancer
and 1981 will claim 420,000 lives. Sex, race, heredity,
geography, age, occupation, economics, habits, and exposure

to substances can contribute significantly to the cause and course of cancer.

Heart disease, the greatest killer stalking the population today, is responsible for over 700,000 deaths each year. Heart disease also causes permanent disability for more workers under 65 years of age than any other illness.

The public's response to a massive awareness campaign about the effects of lifestyle on health precipitated a decline in the incidence of deaths and disabilities due to heart disease and to certain cancers.

ILLNESS AND DISEASE PREVENTION

General

720. Airola, Paavo. HYPOGLYCEMIA: A BETTER APPROACH. Health Plus Publications, Phoenix. 1977.

721. Bennett, Hal, and Samuels, Michael. THE WELL-BODY BOOK. Random House, New York. 1978.

This comprehensive home medical handbook, written by a physician, describes in excellent detail how to do a complete physical exam, how to diagnose common diseases, how to practice preventive medicine, and how to get the most from your doctor. The author includes step-by-step illustrations and an annotated bibliography.

722. Breslow, Lori, ed. HOW TO GET THE BEST HEALTH CARE FOR YOUR MONEY. Rodale Press, Emmaus, Pa. 1979.

This book is a comprehensive guide to new choices in health care. Included are alternatives to using fee-for-service physicians and costly specialists and information on using health maintenance organizations and health care centers.

723. Cahill, Kevin. MEDICAL ADVICE FOR THE TRAVELER. Popular Library, New York. 1977.

This useful book covering all questions involved in traveling includes discussions of innoculations, air sickness, time-zone syndrome, and how to find a physician when overseas. Dr. Cahill offers a medical kit for travelers and discusses food, water, climate, and clothing.

724. Clark, Randolph, and Cumley, Russell W., eds. THE BOOK OF HEALTH. 3rd ed. Van Nostrand Reinhold, New York. 1973.

This authoritative medical encyclopedia is a revised and abridged version of an already popular, comprehensive

medical guide for the family. The book is dedicated to
the principle that a medically informed person receives
the best medical care. Over 270 distinguished specialists have contributed to this book which answers a wide
range of questions on topics of health and disease.

725. Coleman, Lester I. GOOD HOUSEKEEPING ALL YOUR MEDICAL
     QUESTIONS ANSWERED. Hearst Books, New York. 1977.

726. Diekelman, Nancy. PRIMARY HEALTH CARE OF THE WELL
     ADULT. McGraw-Hill, New York. 1977.

This book focuses on the assessment of the primary
health care needs of the well adult, rather than dealing
in any detail with the physical-assessment history and
physical examinations. It offers situations and inter-
ventions that include vignettes of patient-nurse interaction which are designed to help students apply this
new knowledge to nursing care in both primary and
secondary settings.

727. Dong, Collin H., and Banks, Jane. NEW HOPE FOR THE
     ARTHRITIC. Ballantine, Random House, New York. 1976.

The principal author, who has treated thousands of ar-
thritics for 40 years, hypothesizes that the inciting
factors to an arthritic attack are food allergens. The
Dong diet avoids milk products, most meats, and fruits
and fruit juices, as well as common chemical additives.
The book reviews standard treatments of arthritis, contains many case histories, discusses the Dong diet including menus and recipes, and examines the use of acupuncture in arthritis.

728. Finneson, Bernard E., and Freese, Arthur S. THE NEW
     APPROACH TO LOW BACK PAIN. Berkley Publishing, New
     York. 1977.

The authors describe everything you need to know about
your lower back--its problems and their prevention--from
a top neurosurgeon and low back specialist. The book is
a guide to long-range relief for the everyday victim of
this excruciatingly painful condition.

729. Galton, Lawrence. THE COMPLETE BOOK OF SYMPTOMS AND WHAT THEY CAN MEAN. Simon & Schuster, New York. 1978.

This unique book provides a complete guide to more than 350 symptoms and the more than 440 diseases with which they may be associated. Also included are the more than 250 often confusing symptoms that can be caused by modern drugs. In addition, the author lists and describes more than three dozen often-missed diagnoses.

730. Gardner, A. Ward. GOOD HOUSEKEEPING DICTIONARY OF SYMPTOMS. Grosset & Dunlap, New York. 1978.

731. Germann, Donald R. TOO YOUNG TO DIE. Farnsworth, New York. 1974.

732. Goldsmith, Isle. WHY YOU GET SICK AND HOW YOU GET WELL. Sterling Publishing, New York. 1970.

This easy-to-read book, geared to adolescents, is about symptoms, disease, and the medical profession. The text is excellent for health education classes (grades 6 - 10).

733. Goodman, Joseph I. DIABETES WITHOUT FEAR. Avon, New York. 1979.

Separating fact from fiction, the author discloses the latest medical techniques, courses of treatment, and positive scientific realities about diabetes as it relates to marriage, children, diet, complications, insulin, and day-to-day care. The book provides an excellent synthesis of scientific knowledge and personal care.

734. Harper, Harold W., and Culbert, Michael L. HOW YOU CAN BEAT THE KILLER DISEASES. Arlington House, New Rochelle, N.Y. 1978.

735. Katz, Robert S. MEDICAL TESTS YOU CAN DO YOURSELF. Sterling, New York. 1978.

736. Kostrubale, Thaddeus. THE JOY OF RUNNING. Lippincott, New York. 1976.

The author prescribes running as a central therapeutic

technique in his medical practice. He discusses the
specific benefits of running, gives suggestions on food
and clothing, and presents a detailed plan for the
reader, including exercises to do before running.

737. Lipkin, Mack. STRAIGHT TALK ABOUT YOUR HEALTH CARE.
Harper & Row, New York. 1977.

738. Marchetti, Albert. COMMON CURES FOR COMMON AILMENTS.
Stein & Day, Briarcliff Manor, N.Y. 1978.

This valuable home reference book on the use of brand
name medications offers the reader more understanding
and control for healthy living.

739. Miller, Benjamin, and Galton, Lawrence. FAMILY BOOK OF
PREVENTIVE MEDICINE. Simon & Schuster, New York. 1971.

740. Nierenberg, Judith, and Janovic, Florence. THE HOSPITAL
EXPERIENCE. Bobbs-Merrill, Indianapolis. 1978.

There is nothing simple or easy about being sick in the
hospital. It takes months to recover your wits, your
energy, your gaiety, not to mention a sense of physical
well-being. This book will be immensely helpful to
anyone who finds it necessary to cope with the modern
hospital--as patient, relative, or supportive friend.
The authors provide all the advice and encouragement
you need to become an articulate participant in your
own medical care.

741. Nugent, Nancy. HOW TO GET ALONG WITH YOUR STOMACH.
Little, Brown, Boston. 1978.

This commonsense guide rounds out your knowledge of common ailments such as heartburn, indigestion, and ulcers.
The author helps you to discover possible treatments for
the universal complaint of aerophagia ("eating air"),
acid stomach, heartburn, stomach rumblings, and even
hangover. A life-saving chapter outlines easily ef-
fected emergency treatment of "cafe coronary"--choking
on food.

742. Prevention Magazine. THE PREVENTION GUIDE TO SURGERY
AND ITS ALTERNATIVES. Rodale Press, Emmaus, Pa. 1980.

This authoritative guide to surgery combines specific
information on how to avoid the health crises that lead
to surgery and easy-to-follow advice on how to proceed
when surgery is necessary. The book will help the reader to avoid unnecessary surgery, improve the comfort and
outcome of surgery, and sharpen awareness of hospital
costs and insurance.

The reader will learn how to choose a surgeon, how to
talk to him or her, how to get a second opinion, and
how to take advantage of the new and safe alternatives
to surgery.

743. Reuben, David, M.D. THE SAVE YOUR LIFE DIET.
Ballantine, Random House, New York. 1976.

Based on over 600 unassailable articles published in
national and international medical journals, this book
confirms the validity of the findings that a high-fiber
diet has immense positive potential as a powerful tool
of preventive medicine. The author is convinced that
restoring roughage to our daily diet provides protection from cancer of the colon and rectum; ischemic
heart disease; diverticular disease of the colon; appendicitis; phlebitis and resulting blood clots to the
lung; and obesity.

744. Sehnert, Keith W., and Eisenberg, Howard. HOW TO BE
YOUR OWN DOCTOR--SOMETIMES. Grosset & Dunlap, New
York. 1976.

This extremely useful handbook is designed to help
people handle minor illnesses and emergencies without
medical help and major ones without panic. The "Self-
Help Medical Guide" section outlines clearly and in layman's terms symptoms, treatment, and advice on when to
call the doctor for 14 illnesses, 13 injuries, and nine
emergencies.

745. Sontag, Susan.   ILLNESS AS METAPHOR.   Farrar, Straus &
     Giroux, New York.   1978.

     In the past, certain illnesses such as tuberculosis
     symbolized an aesthetic superiority.   This metaphor is
     often reflected currently in our attitudes toward can-
     cer.   The genesis of these metaphors undergo close
     examination in Sontag's book.   Her subject is the un-
     real and often punitive use of illness in our culture.
     Her fundamental point is that illness is not a metaphor,
     and that the most truthful way of regarding illness is
     to resist such metaphoric thinking.

746. Taylor, Robert B.   DR. TAYLOR'S SELF-HELP MEDICAL
     GUIDE.   New American Library, New York.   1978.

747. Walczak, Michael, and Ehrich, Benjamin B.   NUTRITION AND
     WELL-BEING.   Mojave Books, Reseda, Calif.   1977.

     Writing in a clear direct manner, the authors attempt to
     bridge the ever-increasing gap in communications between
     the lab and layperson.   They share with the reader some
     of their international experiences based on current medi-
     cal and biochemical knowledge in the field of nutrition.
     The book stresses two important points: everyone's bio-
     chemical difference and the human system's struggle for
     balance.

748. Zinman, Joseph Aaron.   SECRETS OF HEALTH THAT MANY
     DOCTORS AND DENTISTS MAY NOT KNOW.   Exposition Press,
     Hicksville, N.Y.   1977.

749. Agran, Larry. CANCER CONNECTION: AND WHAT WE CAN DO ABOUT IT. Houghton Mifflin, Boston. 1977.

The cancer connection described in this book is between the disease and the environment. Job-related cancers and cancer risks are documented in rubber, steel, asbestos, dye, woodwork, farm, and petroleum workers, as well as miners, dry cleaners, machinists, smelters, and roofers. The smoking/lung cancer connection, referred to as "cancer for sale," is also included.

750. Culbert, Michael L. FREEDOM FROM CANCER. New ed. Seventy-Six Press, Seal Beach, Calif. 1976.

The controversy over laetrile is referred to as a war. Officialdom's response to laetrile is an included feature, as well as other examples of battles of unorthodoxy in medical lore. Case histories of patients who have been helped--some with complete recoveries--are described in detail.

751. Germann, Donald R., and Danbrot, Margaret. THE ANTI-CANCER DIET. Wideview Books, New York. 1979.

This book offers a diet for protection against cancer, not a cure for the disease. Using the evidence that Seventh Day Adventists, who have special habits of diet and lifestyle, have a lower-than-normal rate of cancer, the authors offer some cancer diet recipes that lack fat, cholesterol, and calories. What fiber can and cannot do is discussed and recipes are offered, from angel food cake to whole wheat pancakes.

752. Kushner, Rose. WHY ME? New American Library, New York. 1977.

The author investigates every aspect of breast cancer, from the scientific to the emotional, the statistical, and the controversial. This extensively researched book provides firsthand information from doctors, researchers, nurses, and breast-cancer patients to help every woman learn to take responsibility for her own safety--and to

find the best possible medical aid should it ever become nessary.

753. Laws, Pricilla. X-RAYS: MORE HARM THAN GOOD? Rodale
     Press, Emmaus, Pa. 1977.

     This book tells how to avoid both the potential health
     risks and the financial burden created by the excessive
     use of X-rays.

754. LeShan, Lawrence. YOU CAN FIGHT FOR YOUR LIFE: EMOTION-
     AL FACTORS IN THE CAUSATION OF CANCER. M. Evans, New
     York. 1977.

     LeShan presents evidence for his unorthodox view that
     cancer patients seem to be a "particular kind of per-
     son." Describing his research that began in the early
     1950s, he suggests that cancer patients have an inabil-
     ity to express anger or resentment and are under emo-
     tional tension surrounding the death of a parent to a
     greater degree than noncancerous individuals. Details
     of the life histories, personality structures based on
     psychological testing, and emotional functioning of
     cancer patients are described.

755. Newbold, H. L. VITAMIN C AGAINST CANCER. Ballantine,
     New York. 1979.

756. Papaioannou, A. N. THE PREVENTION OF BREAST CANCER.
     Warren H. Green, St. Louis, Mo. 1980.

757. Roberts, J. Gordon. CANCER: HOW AND WHY IT MAY BE
     WIPED OUT. Valkyrie Press, St. Petersburg, Fla. 1977.

758. Zalon, Jean. I AM WHOLE AGAIN. Random House, New York,
     1978.

     This book holds out new hope to every woman who has ever
     had breast surgery and allays the concerns of those who
     fear it. The author relates the moving story of one
     woman's search after her mastectomy for the reconstruc-
     tion that would make her feel "whole again."

Prevention of Heart Disease

759. Alpert, Joseph, M.D. THE HEART ATTACK HANDBOOK.
Little, Brown, Boston. 1978.

In clear, everyday terms, the author describes the
physical processes that lead to and characterize a
heart attack, the methods of treatment, and the steps
to recovery. The appendices are invaluable fingertip
references.

760. American Heart Association. THE HEART BOOK. Dutton,
New York. 1979.

761. Bailey, Herbert. VITAMIN E: YOUR KEY TO A HEALTHY
HEART. Arc Books, New York. 1964.

Although this book is over 15 years old, it remains one
of the best sources of information on a controversy
around the usefulness of Vitamin E in preventing heart
disease.

762. Baldry, P. E. THE BATTLE AGAINST HEART DISEASE.
Cambridge University Press, New York. 1971.

This book traces, from the early Greeks to the present
time, the evolution of our knowledge of the principal
diseases of the heart including rheumatic fever, syphilis, bacterial infection of the valves, disturbances
of rate and rhythm, high blood pressure, coronary
thrombosis, and congenital heart disease. It also
describes important advances such as the invention of
cardiac drugs and the development of electrical apparatus for diagnosis and treatment.

763. Blaine, Thomas R. PREVENT THAT HEART ATTACK. Citadel,
Secaucus, N.J. 1972.

The author, a judge with no professional medical background, writes this provocative and well-researched
book and attacks the medical profession for its inep-
titude for not emphasizing the important role of nutrition. He discusses the myths around stress and cholesterol, and the relation of the heart to Vitamins E, C,
and B. Useful appendices are included.

175

764. Cantwell, John D. STAY YOUNG AT HEART. Nelson-Hall,
     Chicago. 1975.

     The book addresses the seemingly healthy person who
     wants to take a closer look at risk factors and tech-
     niques to modify lifestyle for maximum health.

765. Czerwinski, Barbara S. A MANUAL OF PATIENT EDUCATION
     FOR CARDIOPULMONARY DISEASE. C. V. Mosby, St. Louis,
     Mo. 1980.

766. Gerrick, David. ARE YOU A CORONARY CANDIDATE? Dayton
     Labs, Dayton, Ohio. 1978.

767. Jones, Jeanne. DIET FOR A HAPPY HEART. 101 Productions,
     San Francisco. 1975.

     The basic purpose of this useful book is to provide the
     general reader, dieters, and diabetics with appealing
     but perfectly balanced sugar-free recipes for a happy
     heart diet. The menus, applicable to all calorie
     levels, are based on the Diabetic Diet program because
     it is the most frequently prescribed diet for health
     problems. Many famous health spas and the successful
     Weight Watchers program use this diet. The book in-
     cludes instructions on preparing two one-week sample
     menus at two different calorie levels. Each menu
     limits the amount of cholesterol to 200 milligrams per
     day.

768. Kezdi, Paul. YOU AND YOUR HEART. Atheneum, New York.
     1977.

     How does your heart work and what are the causes of
     heart disease? Symptoms, treatment, and research are
     all included in this book on the heart. The importance
     of such factors as sex, heredity, age, physique, emo-
     tions, environment, work, food, drink, sleep, smoking,
     and exercise are all covered, and advice is given on how
     to relax and how to quit smoking.

769. Levitas, Irving, and Machol, Libby. YOU CAN BEAT THE
     ODDS ON HEART ATTACK. Bobbs-Merrill, Indianapolis.
     1976.

770. Lewis, Barry, and Lewis, Eve. THE HEART BOOK: LIVING
     WELL AND TAKING CARE OF YOUR HEART. Barrie & Jenkins,
     New York. 1979.

771. Loughran, John X. NINETY DAYS TO A BETTER HEART. Arc
     Books, New York. 1968.

     This interesting and personal book offers information
     about improving heart efficiency by natural methods.
     The "90-day" campaign is based on the knowledge that
     human red blood cells completely renew themselves every
     30 days, and a 90-day period of intelligent eating and
     living corresponds to about three complete red-blood
     cell renewals. Prebreakfast routine and other circu-
     lation-improving measures are included.

772. Lynch, James J. THE BROKEN HEART. Basic Books, New
     York. 1979.

     The author, a leading specialist in psychosomatic medi-
     cine, shows that the incidence of premature death from
     heart disease is significantly higher among the loneli-
     ness prone--the widowed, divorced, and separated; the
     old and the single young living alone; and children from
     broken homes. He warns that our very physical survival
     is threatened in a society in which the divorce rate is
     rising and the family is fragmenting, and he concludes
     we must learn to live together--or we shall die pre-
     maturely, alone.

773. Maness, William. EXERCISE YOUR HEART. Macmillan,
     New York. 1969.

774. Miller, Robert A. HOW TO LIVE WITH A HEART ATTACK: AND
     HOW TO AVOID ONE. Chilton Book Co., Radnor, Pa. 1978.

     This informative book offers the reader a simplified ex-
     planation of problems to avoid and gives advice on how to
     recognize when medical attention is required for a pos-
     sible heart attack. Dr. Miller wants to help individu-
     als to avoid hurting themselves through ignorance.
     Detailed discussions are provided on such subjects as
     heart attacks, surgery for coronary artery disease,
     heart failure, pacemakers, and pulmonary embolism.

775. Morse, Robert L., ed. EXERCISE AND THE HEART; GUIDE-
     LINES FOR EXERCISE PROGRAMS. Charles C Thomas,
     Springfield, Ill. 1974.

776. Nash, David T. CORONARY: PREDICTION AND PREVENTION.
     Scribner, New York. 1979.

777. Passwater, Richard. SUPERNUTRITION FOR HEALTHY HEARTS:
     THE TOTAL PROTECTION PLAN THROUGH VITAMINS, DIET AND
     EXERCISE. Dial, New York. 1978.

778. Shute, Evan V., and Shute Institute Staff. THE HEART
     AND VITAMIN E. Keats, New Canaan, Conn. 1977.

779. Vineberg, Arthur. HOW TO LIVE WITH YOUR HEART: THE
     FAMILY GUIDE TO HEART HEALTH. Time Books, New York.
     1977.

     This well-illustrated and well-written text for all ages
     offers a program for enjoyment and education. The au-
     thor answers the most common questions and describes the
     biological nature of the heart in detail.

780. Warmbrand, Max. ADD YEARS TO YOUR HEART. BJ Publishing
     Group, New York. 1969.

781. Zohman, Leonore R., Kattus, Albert A., and Softness,
     Donald G. THE CARDIOLOGIST'S GUIDE TO FITNESS AND
     HEALTH THROUGH EXERCISE. Simon & Schuster, New York.
     1979.

     The authors provide a complete understanding of the
     scientific basis of exercise along with excellent refer-
     ence charts, tables, and illustrations. The book helps
     the reader decide whether present physical activity is
     enough or excessive; shows how to devise a personal pro-
     gram; offers ways to fit exercise into time schedules
     and lifestyle; and evaluates exercise programs from
     well-known health clubs and famous spas and appraises a
     variety of exercise systems and equipment.

Cholesterol

782. Cavaiani, Mabel. THE LOW CHOLESTEROL COOKBOOK. Barnes & Noble, New York. 1974.

783. Evans, D. Wainwright, and Greenfield, Meta A., eds. COOKING FOR YOUR HEART'S CONTENT: 250 GOURMET RECIPES TO KEEP YOUR HEART HEALTHY. Paddington Press, New York. 1977.

This book of interesting and easy recipes is designed for people intent on lowering and maintaining low blood cholesterol levels. Recipes most useful to dieters who want to lose weight are clearly marked in the book and a chart provides a quick guide to the more suitable foods.

784. Grace, Vilma J. CHOLESTEROL CONSCIOUS COOKING--THE LATIN WAY: ENTICING INTERNATIONAL RECIPES FROM LATIN AMERICA. Acropolis Books, Washington, D.C. 1979.

The wide variety of Caribbean, Central, and South American dishes presented in this book reflects the author's appreciation of gourmet cookery and her broad knowledge of the principles of good nutrition.

785. Kaufman, William I. BRAND NAME GUIDE TO CALORIES AND CARBOHYDRATES. BJ Publishing, New York. 1975.

786. Kaufman, William I. GUIDE TO CHOLESTEROL. Baronet, New York. 1978.

787. Kraus, Barbara. DICTIONARY OF SODIUM, FATS AND CHOLESTEROL. Grosset & Dunlap, New York. 1974.

The author, a foremost health and nutrition expert, has compiled thousands of food items and calculated their sodium, fat, and cholesterol content based on United States Department of Agriculture data and information from manufacturers and processors. Portion sizes are taken into account, eliminating guesswork in calculating undesirable ingredients in just about everything we eat.

788. Leviton, Roberta. THE JEWISH LOW-CHOLESTEROL COOKBOOK.
     Paul S. Eriksson, Middlebury, Vt. 1978.

     Over 200 traditional kosher recipes, including borscht
     and chicken soup, are included in this cookbook which
     is designed to help the reader avoid cholesterol in the
     diet. The medical rationale for the recipes is de-
     scribed as well as some basic principles of low-choles-
     terol cooking.

789. McFarlane, Helen B. THE CHOLESTEROL CONTROL COOKBOOK.
     Baronet, New York. 1977.

     This handy book of simple, easy-to-follow recipes
     stresses balance, variety, and small or moderate help-
     ings of food as the key to controlling cholesterol
     levels as well as many chronic or acute disabilities.

790. Revell, Dorothy. CHOLESTEROL CONTROL COOKERY. Berkley
     Publishing, New York. 1973.

     These saturated fat-free recipes bring variety to food
     preparation. A listing of the foods "used" and
     "avoided" on this modified fat diet is included as an
     aid to meal planning. The author includes the basic
     seven food groups in the daily menus.

791. Roth, June. LOW-CHOLESTEROL JEWISH COOKERY: THE
     UNSATURATED FAT WAY. Arco, New York. 1978.

     Even change of lifestyle for health purposes is trau-
     matic. Such change is especially difficult when tamper-
     ing with Jewish delectables. The author takes the
     challenge--successfully--of removing the "chicken fat"
     from the preparation of Jewish foods and provides the
     opportunity to eat and live well.

792. Wade, Carlson. FACT-BOOK ON FATS, OILS AND CHOLESTEROL.
     Keats, New Canaan, Conn. 1973.

     This practical book offers facts on animal and vegetable
     fats, oils, and cholesterol. Advice is offered on how
     to select meats to avoid fat. Doctor-tested menus and
     recipes are provided.

793. Weiss, Elizabeth, and Wolfson, Rita P. THE GOURMET'S
     LOW-CHOLESTEROL COOKBOOK. BJ Publishing Group, New
     York. 1974.

     The book outlines some of the information known about
     the relation between diet and atherosclerosis. The
     author explains why the American Heart Association,
     other reputable foundations, most physicians, and
     nutritionists recommend a low-cholesterol, low-saturat-
     ed fat eating plan for all average healthy Americans.

794. Zane, Polly. THE JACK SPRAT COOKBOOK, OR GOOD EATING
     ON A LOW-CHOLESTEROL DIET. Harper & Row, New York.
     1973.

     This excellent book provides palatable, interesting,
     and even exciting meals for most patients with choles-
     terol problems. The author, faced with the practical
     problem of providing her husband with a diet low in
     saturated fat and cholesterol, has managed to use her
     considerable imagination to adapt recipes and cooking
     techniques to meet this goal.

795. Allen, William A.; Angerman, G.; and Fackler, W. A.
LEARNING TO LIVE WITHOUT CIGARETTES. Doubleday,
New York. 1968.

In Section I of this book, specific suggestions are offered to rid the smoker of a dependence on cigarettes.
The latest information and insights on the peculiarities
of the cigarette habit are examined. Section II provides the professional worker with specific anti-
smoking activities for use in community settings.

796. Bellino, Robert J. SMOKE-OUT. Anthelion Press,
Corte Madera, Calif. 1979.

797. Brean, Herbert. HOW TO STOP SMOKING. Rev. ed. Pocket
Books, New York. 1975.

This book offers the reader a practical guide to ending
the habit. Helpful day-by-day observations and advice
add extra support for the first two weeks of cessation.

798. Burton, D., and Wohl, Gary S. JOY OF QUITTING: HOW TO
HELP YOUNG PEOPLE STOP SMOKING. Macmillan, New York.
1979.

Young people start smoking to be "cool." This book explains what "being cool" does to their bodies. Joy
of Quitting is addressed to all young people who smoke
and to those who want to help them quit. The authors
offer the reader facts about smoking in clear, non-
alarmist language, explaining reasons young people smoke
and why, after a period, so many are ready to quit.
Simple, sensible steps to quit the habit are offered.

799. Chesser, Eustace. DO YOU WANT TO STOP SMOKING?
Cornerstone Library, New York. 1976.

800. Colby, Anthony O. A DOCTOR'S BOOK ON SMOKING AND HOW TO
QUIT. Contemporary Books, Chicago. 1978.

Dr. Colby, who smoked four packs a day for 15 years, offers practical advice to help smokers give up the habit.
He discusses the history of smoking, medical evidence

against smoking, and the effects of smoking on a person's energy level, sex, and senses. Also provided
are a daily menu guide to keep blood pressure and weight
down and a simple exercise program to stay fit.

801. Danaher, Brian G., and Lichtenstein, Edward. BECOME AN
EX-SMOKER. Prentice-Hall, Englewood Cliffs, N.J. 1978.

This self-help workbook is divided into two major parts:
a discussion of skills necessary for becoming an ex-
smoker and the listing of a resource appendix on smoking
issues. The authors have designed the program to help
cope with and eliminate the lingering smoking urges that
would cause a fledgling ex-smoker to resume the habit.

802. De Mente, Boye. KICKING THE SMOKING HABIT. Phoenix
Books, Phoenix. 1978.

803. Diehl, Harold S. TOBACCO AND YOUR HEALTH: THE SMOKING
CONTROVERSY. McGraw-Hill, New York. 1969.

This book presents scientific and medically accepted information and judgment on this subject. The author
frankly disclaims the roles of disinterested observer
and impartial reporter as he discusses tobacco and
health because, as Dean of Medical Science and Professor of Public Health at the University of Minnesota, he
has "seen too much illness, disability and premature
death attributable to smoking" to remain impartial.
Despite the emotional involvement, this is a scientific
book.

804. Doron, Gideon. THE SMOKING PARADOX: PUBLIC REGULATION
IN THE CIGARETTE INDUSTRY. Abt Associates, Cambridge,
Mass. 1979.

Professor Doron's analysis of the regulatory action in
the cigarette industry shows how misleading are the pre-
suppositions which underlie these actions--the presuppo-
sitions that the force of government can make people
better human beings and how this force can bring about
a desired state of affairs. This study adds one more
piece to the swiftly growing body of evidence that, con-
trary to the sentimental and simple-minded expectations

of reformers, society cannot easily enforce goodness,
nor can social outcomes be changed by fact.

805. DuCharme, Diane; Angel-Levy, P.; and Mitz, R. THE
     CIGARETTE PAPERS: SNIP THE STRINGS TO YOUR HABIT.
     CompCare, Minneapolis. 1979.

806. Edwards, Griffith; Hawks, David; Russell, Michael; and
     MacCafferty, Maxine. ALCOHOL DEPENDENCE AND SMOKING
     BEHAVIOR. Lexington Books, Lexington, Mass. 1976.

807. Geisinger, David L. KICKING IT: THE NEW WAY TO STOP
     SMOKING PERMANENTLY. Grove, New York. 1979.

     The key word in this approach to quitting smoking is
     "permanently." Dr. Geisinger presents his five-week
     program for quitting and follows it up with graduate
     and post-graduate advice. Weapons against oral craving,
     eating, weight gain, and the influence of other smokers
     are offered, and exercises and new habit patterns for
     permanent resistance to smoking are suggested.

808. Harris, Roger W. HOW TO KEEP ON SMOKING AND LIVE.
     St. Martin's, New York. 1978.

     This different kind of book is written in a light and
     humorous way by a serious cigarette smoker who guaran-
     tees a 90% reduction in tar and nicotine while still
     enjoying the same amount of cigarette smoking.

809. Hull, Clark L. THE INFLUENCE OF TOBACCO SMOKING ON
     MENTAL AND MOTOR EFFICIENCY. Greenwood Press, Westport,
     Conn. 1975.

     This volume represents the results of a study of the re-
     lation of tobacco to mental efficiency. The author sum-
     marizes the results of previous investigations and
     discusses the methods employed to secure reliable data.

810. Hyde, Margaret O. ADDICTIONS. McGraw-Hill, New York.
     1978.

     The author does a competent job of analyzing addictions,
     e.g., cigarette, gambling, coffee, drugs, and jogging
     and offers methods of cessation or control such as

relaxation, deep breathing, behavioral contracting, ex-smoker witness, buddy system, and group therapy.

811. Madison, Arnold. SMOKING AND YOU. Messner, New York. 1975.

This book is designed for use by elementary school children. It examines biological function, the smoking habit, and other issues that may help prevent children from smoking.

812. Marr, John S. A BREATH OF AIR AND A BREATH OF SMOKE (Gr. 3 - 6). M. Evans, New York. 1971.

813. Matchan, Don C. WE MIND IF YOU SMOKE. BJ Publishing Group, New York. 1977.

814. McKean, Margaret. THE STOP SMOKING BOOK. Impact Publishers, San Luis Obispo, Calif. 1976.

815. Michaelsen, James A. HOW YOU CAN STOP SMOKING NOW: AS I DID AFTER THIRTY-THREE YEARS. Exposition Press, Hicksville, N.Y. 1979.

816. Rogers, Jacqueline. YOU CAN STOP: THE SMOKENDERS GUIDE ON HOW TO GIVE UP CIGARETTES. Pocket Books, New York. 1979.

A practical manual designed to bridge the gap between just wanting to try to quit smoking and the actual motivation needed for success, this book presents a psychological approach to quitting. Hunches are offered on why people smoke and what to say to someone you love who smokes.

817. Ross, Walter S. YOU CAN QUIT SMOKING IN 14 DAYS. Berkley Publishing, New York. 1976.

This reassuring book provides an easy-to-live-with 14-day program for cigarette smokers who want to give up the habit. Proven quitting aids are described along with sound advice from ex-smokers on how they did it. Since most smokers are motivated to give up cigarettes for health reasons, the book also highlights the latest

research on the hazards of smoking and the benefits
of quitting.

818. Sobel, Robert. THEY SATISFY: THE CIGARETTE IN AMERICAN
LIFE. Doubleday, New York. 1978.

This well-researched book presents both sides of the
coin objectively and engages the reader in a forth-
right discussion of the cigarette/cancer controversy.

819. Stewart, Maxwell S. CIGARETTES: AMERICA'S NO. 1 HEALTH
PROBLEM. Rev. ed. Public Affairs Com., New York.
1972.

820. Worick, W., and Schaller, W. ALCOHOL, TOBACCO AND
DRUGS: THEIR USE AND ABUSE. Prentice-Hall, Englewood
Cliffs, N.J. 1977.

The central theme of this college-level book stresses
the importance of education and prevention in dealing
with problems associated with alcohol, tobacco, and
drugs. The authors state that failure to grapple with
these problems represents a betrayal to society. An
innovative separate chapter addressing some of the
basic issues on theories of dependence helps to broaden
the reader's perspective and understanding.

821. Barlow, David. SEXUALLY TRANSMITTED DISEASES: THE FACTS.
     Oxford University Press, New York. 1979.

     This well-illustrated and comprehensive text does not
     limit itself only to a discussion of syphilis and gon-
     orrhea but includes many other venereal diseases such
     as chancroid, non-specific genital infections, herpes
     genitales, and trichomoniases.

822. Blanzaco, Andre. VD: FACTS YOU SHOULD KNOW. (Gr. 7 -
     12). Lothrop, New York. 1970.

823. Brooks, Stewart M. THE V.D. STORY. A.S. Barnes,
     Cranbury, N.J. 1971.

     This book presents the interested general reader with
     the highlights of this subject. Helpful illustrations
     and drawings facilitate understanding.

824. Chiappa, Joseph, and Forish, Joseph J. THE VD BOOK.
     Holt, Rinehart & Winston, New York. 1977.

     This is the official publication of the U. S. Alliance
     for the Eradication of Veneral Disease. Common ques-
     tions and answers on what VD is, the difference between
     syphilis and other diseases, and how VD happens are in-
     cluded.

825. Johnson, Eric W. V.D.: VENEREAL DISEASE AND WHAT YOU
     SHOULD DO ABOUT IT   (Gr. 5 - 12). New rev. ed.
     Lippincott, New York. 1978.

826. Klingbeil, Reinhold. VD IS NOT FOR ME. Southern
     Publishing, Nashville, Tenn. 1976.

827. Lasagna, Louis. THE VD EPIDEMIC: HOW IT STARTED, WHERE
     IT'S GOING AND WHAT TO DO ABOUT IT. Temple University
     Press, Philadelphia. 1975.

     The question of what brought about the epidemic of VD in
     the 1960's and 1970's is thoroughly probed in this
     straightforward book. The symptoms, source, and conse-
     quences of VD, as well as effective therapy therefor are

described in an attempt to expose past hypocrisy and to dispel present ignorance on this subject.

828. Llewellyn-Jones, Derek. SEX AND VD. Merrimack Book Service, Bridgeport, Conn. 1975.

A very easy-to-read book which covers historical, social, and biological aspects of V.D.

829. Morton, Barbara M. V.D.: A GUIDE FOR NURSES AND COUNSELORS. Little, Brown, Boston. 1976.

830. Nicholas, Leslie. HOW TO AVOID SOCIAL DISEASES: A HANDBOOK. Stein & Day, Briarcliff Manor, N.Y. 1973.

Written in the form of questions and answers, this non-technical book provides proven scientific facts about venereal diseases and discusses the results of many physicians' experiences in language that neither confuses nor belittles the reader.

831. Rosebury, Theodor. MICROBES AND MORALS. Ballantine, New York. 1976.

The word "morals" in the title refers broadly to those aspects of venereal disease that are relevant to matters of human behavior. Under the section on microbes, and well within the grasp of the general reader, the author addresses the many technical aspects of V.D. This book is also an excellent source for those interested in the history and social aspects of venereal disease.

832. Stein, Mari. VD: THE LOVE EPIDEMIC. Rev. ed. Quarterdeck Press, Pacific Palisades, Calif. 1977.

Through imaginative cartoons and straightforward explanation, the author provides parents and other interested individuals with an easy way to discuss a tough subject. These cartoons are an excellent medium for an easy understanding of the aspects of gonorrhea, syphilis, and myths about V.D. The book includes a V.D. Hall of Fame among whose members are Hitler, Van Gogh, and Nietzsche.

833. Young, Eleanor R. VENEREAL DISEASE (Gr. 7 - 12). Watts, New York. 1973.

MENTAL HEALTH

For over 350 years society had banished the mentally
ill to custodial institutions where the census increased
yearly and few were discharged. Psychiatrists functioned
mainly as administrators and custodians. The situation
was exacerbated by public apathy, social stigma, and the
lack of knowledge of effective treatment.

In the past 20 years this practice has been dramatically reversed by pharmacology. The discovery of drugs
for suppressing the symptoms of many mental disorders
returned patients to their communities. The psychiatric
profession agreed that ongoing treatment in the local
community was likely to be more effective in many instances
than warehousing the mentally disturbed in large remote
asylums. Pharmacological agents alone were not responsible
for the dramatic changes in the treatment of mentally ill
patients.

At the end of World War II, the country shifted to a
predominantly urban, technological society accompanied by
changes in long-standing beliefs and traditions. The
stress of accelerated social change generated a national
focus on the mental health of the country. Psychological
insights gained during wartime from soldiers unable to
perform in battle, and the psychological problems experienced by returning veterans heralded the evolution of the
mental health movement.

Gradually a set of useful therapies emerged: crisis
intervention, brief psychotherapy, group therapy, family
therapy, community therapy, and behavior modification. The
spirit of social reform prevalent in the 1960s led to the
establishment of community mental health centers. The
pursuit of mental health became a national pasttime. An
abundance of funds made psychiatry and psychology not only
legitimate but fashionable. Interest in mental health
infiltrated every area of society.

Today, the mental health field not only grapples with
self-actualization and self-fulfillment, but it also de-
termines what populations require services, what services

189

are to be delivered, and what professional groups should
provide the services.

The next decade will see mental health moving to a
closer integration with medicine to consolidate the search
for new methods to relieve the emotional burdens of life
in a complex society.

MENTAL HEALTH

General

834. Allen, Richard, ed. MENTAL HEALTH IN AMERICA: THE
YEAR OF CRISIS. Marquis, Chicago. 1979.

835. Allen, Robert, and Cartier, Marsha. THE MENTAL HEALTH
ALMANAC. New ed. Garland, New York. 1978-79.

This book is an excellent resource guide to the field
of mental health. The text is divided into three sections: the population requiring services, the concern
for delivering services, and the professional group to
provide them. Each section contains a pertinent list
of books, articles, audio tapes, and films.

836. Amada, Gerald. MENTAL HEALTH AND AUTHORITARIANISM ON
THE COLLEGE CAMPUS. University Press of America,
Washington, D.C. 1979.

837. Amary, Issam B. THE RIGHTS OF THE MENTALLY RETARDED--
DEVELOPMENTALLY DISABLED TO TREATMENT AND EDUCATION.
Charles C Thomas, Springfield, Ill. 1979.

This book presents a summary of the current legal developments in the field of mental health and provides a
starting point for any individual who wishes to become
acquainted with the broad changes taking place.

838. Bisch, Louis E. CURE YOUR NERVES YOURSELF. Rev. ed.
Fawcett, New York. 1977.

839. Bry, Adelaide. GETTING BETTER. Rawson Wade, New York.
1979.

840. Burgum, Thomas, and Anderson, Scott. THE COUNSELOR AND
THE LAW. American Personnel and Guidance Assn.
Washington, D.C. 1975.

This book examines the law as it relates to counseling
services. Potential malpractice problems associated
with birth control, abortion, drug or illegal search,
confidentiality, libel, or outright criminality are
discussed. This volume can help counselors because the
text is written by lawyers who understand counseling.

841. Burrow, Trigent. A SEARCH FOR MAN'S SANITY. Arno,
     New York. 1979.

842. Cahow, Clark R. PEOPLE, PATIENTS AND POLITICS. Arno,
     New York. 1979.

843. Chen, Peter W. CHINESE-AMERICANS VIEW THEIR MENTAL
     HEALTH. R&E Research Associates, Palo Alto, Calif.
     1977.

844. Chesler, Phyllis. WOMEN AND MADNESS. Avon, New York.
     1973.

     This book is about dramatically increasing numbers of
     American women who are seen or who see themselves as
     "neurotic" or "psychotic" and who seek help and/or are
     hospitalized. The author answers questions about be-
     havior and describes what happens to a person in need of
     help and how this help is or is not forthcoming.

845. Chu, Franklin, and Trotter, Sharland. THE MADNESS
     ESTABLISHMENT: RALPH NADER'S STUDY GROUP REPORT ON THE
     NATIONAL INSTITUTE OF MENTAL HEALTH. Viking, New York.
     1974.

846. Coan, Richard N. HERO, ARTIST, SAGE OR SAINT? Columbia
     University Press, New York. 1977.

     This volume is a survey of views on what is variously
     called mental health, normality, maturity, self-
     actualization, and human fulfillment.

847. Cosgrove, Mark P., and Schmidt, Marty. ESSENCE OF HUMAN
     NATURE. Zondervan Publ., Grand Rapids, Mich. 1977.

     This book examines current evidence from psychological
     research and emphasizes the inadequacy of those views
     which describe man as just a materialistic, totally

deterministic higher animal. The authors critically
evaluate the deterministic model of B. F. Skinner,
language studies in chimpanzees, and recent brain control experiments.

848. Craig, Paul. MY LOOK AT LIFE ITSELF. Vantage, New
York. 1973.

849. David, Henry P., ed. CHILD MENTAL HEALTH IN INTER-
NATIONAL PERSPECTIVE. Harper & Row, New York. 1972.

This book offers an international perspective to deal
with the perplexing problems of disturbed, delinquent,
retarded, and culturally disadvantaged youths in the
U. S. The authors focus on the organization and delivery of services, and suggest innovations in group
care, manpower utilization, and prevention.

850. Deutsch, Albert, ed. ENCYCLOPEDIA OF MENTAL HEALTH.
2nd printing. Scarecrow Press, Metuchen, N.J. 1970.

851. Dudley, Donald M., and Walke, Elton. HOW TO SURVIVE
BEING ALIVE. New American Library, New York. 1979.

852. Dyer, Wayne W. YOUR ERRONEOUS ZONES. Avon, New York.
1977.

A practicing therapist and counselor, Dr. Dyer relates
his own remarkable success story while writing a very
practical, self-actualization book.

853. Fabricant, Benjamin; Krasner, Jack D.; and Barron,
Jules. TO ENJOY IS TO LIVE: PSYCHOTHERAPY EXPLAINED.
Nelson-Hall, Chicago. 1977.

854. Fast, Julius. CREATIVE COPING: A GUIDE TO POSITIVE
LIVING. Wm. Morrow, New York. 1976.

855. Fensterheim, Herbert. HELP WITHOUT PSYCHO-ANALYSIS.
Stein & Day, New York. 1975.

This book tells what behavior therapy is and what it
can do for the individual who wants a proven shortcut
for solving problems.

856. Finney, Joseph. CULTURE CHANGE, MENTAL HEALTH AND
     POVERTY. Simon & Schuster, New York. 1970.

857. Fisher, Seymour, and Cleveland, Sidney. BODY IMAGE AND
     PERSONALITY. Rev. ed. Dover, New York. 1968.

     This revised and expanded edition examines some of the
     nearly 125 dissertations and studies that have been
     undertaken on the subject since 1958. The authors were
     the first to explore in depth the influence of an indi-
     vidual's concept of his own body (body image) on his
     behavior.

858. Gary, Lawrence E., ed. MENTAL HEALTH: A CHALLENGE TO
     THE BLACK COMMUNITY. Dorrance, Ardmore, Pa. 1978.

859. Gilbert, Jeanne G., and Sullivan, Catherine M. THE
     MENTAL HEALTH AIDE. Springer, New York. 1976.

860. Gladstone, William. TEST YOUR OWN MENTAL HEALTH. New
     American Library, New York. 1979.

     This book is an invaluable diagnostic aid for people who
     want to evaluate their own mental health and learn to
     spot possible danger signals in the behavior of close
     friends and loved ones. The use of specially devised
     diagnostic checklists enables the reader to score his
     or her own behavior in seven revealing areas.

861. Goldberg, Joan, and Hymowitz, Ellen. MENTAL HEALTH
     ACTIVITIES IN THE CLASSROOM: A HANDBOOK. Western
     Psychological Services, Los Angeles. 1977.

862. Griffin, J. D.; Laycock, S. R.; and Line, W. MENTAL
     HYGIENE: A MANUAL FOR TEACHERS. Arden Library, Darby,
     Pa. 1978.

863. Gurin, Gerald, and Veroff, Joseph. AMERICANS VIEW THEIR
     MENTAL HEALTH. Arno, New York. 1979.

864. Harris, Thomas. I'M OK--YOU'RE OK. Avon, New York.
     1976.

     This best seller is the product of Dr. Harris' pioneer-
     ing efforts in the field of transactional analysis--

efforts that have revolutionized therapy procedures
throughout the world. The author translates startling
theories into easily understood language and adapts key
ingredients of successful behavior change into practical
advice.

865. Helmering, Doris Wild. GROUP THERAPY, WHO NEEDS IT?
     Celestial Arts, Millbrae, Calif. 1976.

     The author, an experienced group leader, discusses the
     reasons people come to therapy groups, the variety of
     problems they bring, the indications that small problems
     often signify larger ones, the ways in which people
     sabotage themselves, the myth that therapists are gods,
     and the method of selecting a therapist. A book that
     answers those questions that you might be afraid to ask.

866. Jones, Kenneth L.; Shainberg, Louis W.; and Byer, Curtis
     O. EMOTIONAL HEALTH. 2nd ed. Harper & Row, New York.
     1975.

867. Just, Marion; Bell, Carolyn Shaw; Fisher, Walter; and
     Schensul, Stephen L. COPING IN A TROUBLED SOCIETY.
     Lexington Books, Lexington, Mass. 1974.

     A portion of this book evolved from a study conference
     on "The Future of Mental Health," held in January 1974,
     under the sponsorship of the National Institute of
     Mental Health (NIMH) and San Francisco State College.
     This volume represents considerable rethinking and exten-
     sive revision from previously held conventional wisdoms.
     Specially significant chapters are: "A Sane Economy for
     a Sane People," "Coping with Political Alienation,"
     "Toward Community-Oriented Mental Health Services," and
     "Treatment through Institutional Change." The first and
     last chapters in this volume discuss the environmental
     approach to mental health and the current orientation of
     mental health policies.

868. Kellam, Sheppard G.; Branch, Jeanette D.; Agrawal,
     Khazan C.; and Ensminger, Margaret E. MENTAL HEALTH AND
     GOING TO SCHOOL. University of Chicago Press, Chicago.
     1975.

869. Keyes, Fenton. YOUR FUTURE IN A MENTAL HEALTH CENTER.
     Rosen Press, New York. 1979.

     This book examines opportunities for a career in the
     field of mental health. The author explores personal-
     ities, abilities, and education necessary for a career
     decision and examines geographical locations, attitudes,
     and community mental health centers.

870. Kornhauser, Arthur. MENTAL HEALTH OF THE INDUSTRIAL
     WORKER: A DETROIT STUDY. Krieger, Huntington, N.Y.
     1975.

871. Libo, Lester. IS THERE LIFE AFTER GROUP? HOW TO SELECT,
     SURVIVE AND EXPAND THE ENCOUNTER GROUP EXPERIENCE.
     Anchor Press (Doubleday), New York. 1977.

     With so much conflicting information already written
     about encounter groups, Lester Libo's book is a welcome
     beacon of sane good sense. It should be equally bene-
     ficial reading for those who have had group therapy or
     for anyone planning to join a group either as a partici-
     pant or leader.

872. Masters, Roy. HOW YOUR MIND CAN KEEP YOU WELL. Rev. ed.
     Fawcett, New York. 1977.

873. May, Gerald G. SIMPLY SANE. G. K. Hall, Boston. 1977.

874. Miller, Donald. BODYMIND: THE WHOLE PERSON HEALTH BOOK.
     Prentice-Hall, Englewood Cliffs, N.J. 1974.

875. Mishara, Brian, and Patterson, Robert. CONSUMER'S HAND-
     BOOK OF MENTAL HEALTH: HOW TO FIND, SELECT, AND USE HELP.
     New American Library, New York. 1979.

876. Morgan, Arthur J., and Johnston, Mabyl K. MENTAL HEALTH
     AND MENTAL ILLNESS. 2nd ed. Lippincott, New York. 1976.

877. Myerson, Abraham. INHERITANCE OF MENTAL DISEASES.
     Arno, New York. 1976.

     This book discusses various theories of the "heredity"
     of mental diseases and shows how the term insanity is a
     hindrance to the proper understanding of mental disease.

878. Norback, Judith. MENTAL HEALTH YEARBOOK AND DIRECTORY.
NINETEEN SEVENTY NINE TO NINETEEN EIGHTY. Van Nostrand
Reinhold, New York. 1979.

879. Park, Clara C., and Shapiro, Leon N. YOU ARE NOT ALONE:
UNDERSTANDING AND DEALING WITH MENTAL ILLNESS. Little,
Brown, Boston. 1979.

880. Polenz, Donald G. HELPING AS A HUMANISTIC PROCESS:
PERSPECTIVES AND VIEWPOINTS. University Press of
America, Washington, D.C. 1976.

881. Pothier, Patricia C. MENTAL HEALTH COUNSELING WITH
CHILDREN: A GUIDE FOR BEGINNING COUNSELORS. Little,
Brown, Boston. 1976.

882. Ruitenbeek, Hendrik M. THE NEW GROUP THERAPIES. Avon,
New York. 1970.

This handbook explores the evolution, achievements,
methods, and organization of virtually all the new
psychotherapeutic movements since the relinquishing of
traditional doctor-patient privacy to the acceptance of
self-revelation through mutual confrontation. The
author acquaints the reader with many esoteric therapies
from psychodrama to sensitivity groups, from Synanon and
Daytop to the Esalen experiment, from nude happenings to
marathon encounters, and more. Dr. Ruitenbeek discusses
how people learn to experience the impact they make on
one another.

883. Schwab, John J. SOCIAL ORDER AND MENTAL HEALTH: THE
FLORIDA HEALTH STUDY. Brunner-Mazel, New York. 1979.

884. Shneour, Elie A. THE MALNOURISHED MIND. Doubleday,
New York. 1974.

This book reviews pertinent material on early-life malnutrition and the consequences on human cognition. Although the author is not an alarmist, he presents some
startling facts and formulations that have implications
to the future of civilization.

885. Valletutti, P. PREVENTING PHYSICAL AND MENTAL
DISABILITIES. University Park Press, Baltimore. 1979.

886. Wesley, Roland. ASPECTS OF MENTAL HEALTH: A GUIDE TO
     UNDERSTANDING THE MEANING OF MENTAL ILLNESS. Carlinshar,
     Bolingbrook, Ill. 1979.

     This book provides the layreader with basic ideas about
     civil liberties, mental illness, mental retardation, and
     the processes involved in their causation, prevention,
     control, and treatment.

887. Wilson, John P. THE RIGHTS OF ADOLESCENTS IN THE MENTAL
     HEALTH SYSTEM. Lexington Books, Lexington, Mass. 1978.

Depression

888. Anthony, E. James, and Benedek, Therese, eds. DEPRESSION
AND HUMAN EXISTENCE. Little, Brown, Boston. 1975.

889. Arieti, Silvano, and Bemporad, Jules. SEVERE AND MILD
DEPRESSION. Basic Books, New York. 1978.

890. Barrett, Roger K. DEPRESSION--WHAT IT IS AND WHAT TO DO
ABOUT IT. Cook Publishing, Elgin, Ill. 1977.

The author presents a sensitive and thorough discussion
of the experience of depression, childhood determinants
of depression, the role of anger, inferiority feelings,
and guilt. The book shows how one can cope with depression based on Christian beliefs and ideologies.

891. Benson, George A. WHAT TO DO WHEN YOU'RE DEPRESSED:
A CHRISTIAN PSYCHOANALYST HELPS YOU UNDERSTAND AND OVER-
COME YOUR DEPRESSION. Augsburg Publishing House,
Minneapolis. 1975.

892. Brown, George W., and Harris, Tirril. SOCIAL ORIGINS
OF DEPRESSION: A STUDY OF PSYCHIATRIC DISORDER IN WOMEN.
Free Press, New York. 1978.

A well-documented study of clinical depression as it
relates to women.

893. Buck, Peggy S. I'M DEPRESSED--ARE YOU LISTENING, LORD?
Judson Press, Valley Forge, Pa. 1978.

894. Deffner, Donald L. YOU SAY YOU'RE DEPRESSED. Abingdon
Press, Nashville, Tenn. 1976.

The author contends that an antidote to an unhappy life
is inspiration, and he attempts to show the reader how
to live each moment to the fullest by putting more of
God into daily life.

895. De Rosis, Helen, and Pellegrino, Victoria Y. THE BOOK OF
HOPE: HOW WOMEN CAN OVERCOME DEPRESSION. Macmillan, New
York. 1976.

This book tries to help the reader understand the

phenomenon of anxiety with the hope that its fearful, incapacitating aspect will be diminished. The authors have developed a 20-step program to harness stress and show many examples of women who have learned to use anxiety as a "handle" for identifying trouble points.

896. Flach, Frederic F. THE SECRET STRENGTH OF DEPRESSION. Bantam, New York. 1975.

The author, using case studies, delves into the nature of depression, the opportunity for change, and the recognition of depression. The reader learns the bio-logical basis for depression, and what can be expected of psychotherapy.

897. Galton, Lawrence. THE BODY RULES. Simon & Schuster, New York. 1979.

898. Hampton, Russell K. THE FAR SIDE OF DESPAIR: A PERSONAL ACCOUNT OF DEPRESSION. Nelson-Hall, Chicago. 1975.

899. Kiev, Ari. THE COURAGE TO LIVE. T. Y. Crowell, New York. 1979.

900. Kline, Nathan. FROM SAD TO GLAD: KLINE ON DEPRESSION. Putnam, New York. 1974.

901. Knauth, Percy. A SEASON IN HELL. Harper & Row, New York. 1975.

The author, a successful writer, relates how he turned his suicidal depression into a very positive life force which enabled him to live life much more deeply than before.

902. Kraines, Samuel H., and Thetford, Eloise S. HELP FOR THE DEPRESSED. Charles C Thomas, Springfield, Ill. 1979.

903. La Haye, Tim. HOW TO WIN OVER DEPRESSION. Bantam, New York. 1976.

904. Larsen, Earnest. HOW TO UNDERSTAND AND OVERCOME DEPRESSION. Liguori Publ., Liguori, Mo. 1977.

Larsen's book focuses on the psychological cause and
the spiritual solution to overcoming depression.

905. Lewinsohn, Peter; Munoz, Richard F.; Youngren, Maryann;
and Zeis, Antonette. CONTROL YOUR DEPRESSION. Prentice-
Hall, Englewood Cliffs, N.J. 1978.

906. Lowry, Michael R. PREVENTING MENTAL DEPRESSION. Green,
St. Louis, Mo. 1980.

907. Roth, June. THE FOOD-DEPRESSION CONNECTION.
Contemporary Books, Chicago. 1979.

This practical, down-to-earth book about food allergies
concentrates on the day-to-day problems of providing
adequate nutrition while circumventing specific food
sensitivities.

908. Seligman, Martin E. HELPLESSNESS: ON DEPRESSION,
DEVELOPMENT AND DEATH. W. H. Freeman, San Francisco.
1975.

This excellent resource attempts to analyze the many
aspects of human helplessness by applying theory and
relevant knowledge from the laboratory.

909. Sturgeon, Wina. DEPRESSION: HOW TO RECOGNIZE IT, HOW
TO CURE IT AND HOW TO GAIN FROM IT. Prentice-Hall,
Englewood Cliffs, N.J. 1979.

This book reports the results of ten years' research on
depression, which the author considers to be one of the
most widespread and most insidious diseases ever to afflict mankind. The book tells the reader what depression is and how it can be treated. It offers constructive methods to prevent attacks of depression and
explains where to find help.

910. Wright, Helen D. RELIEF FROM DEPRESSION. Price, Stern,
Sloan, Los Angeles. 1978.

911. Wright, Norman. LIVING WITH YOUR EMOTIONS: SELF-IMAGE
AND DEPRESSION. Harvest House, Irvine, Calif. 1979.

912. Yarbrough, Tom. HOW TO BE HAPPY WITH YOURSELF: A
     GUIDE TO OVERCOME DEPRESSION AND FAILURE. Libra,
     Roslyn Heights, N.Y. 1975.

     The main purpose of this work is to help the reader ac-
     quire the necessary tools for problem solving. Includ-
     ed are suggestions about money, family, and self-
     fulfillment. The author makes suggestions for better
     comprehension of value systems and offers means to ac-
     complish desired goals.

913. Anderson, Robert A. STRESS POWER: HOW TO TURN TENSION
INTO ENERGY. Human Science Press, New York. 1978.

The physician/author charts the precise ways that
stress affects the body and mind and guides the reader
to make stress a positive rather than negative power in
life. Techniques of relaxation, self-awareness, behavior modification, and growth are explained.

914. Benjamin, Ben E. ARE YOU TENSE? THE BENJAMIN SYSTEM
OF MUSCULAR THERAPY. Pantheon, New York. 1978.

This handsome, well-illustrated book offers exercises
for most parts of the body—eyes, jaws, neck, arm and
hand, shoulder, lower back, and legs and feet. General
body care and the use of drugs are discussed, and warm-
up exercises for runners, dancers, and athletes are
included.

915. Benson, Herbert. THE RELAXATION RESPONSE. G. K. Hall,
New York. 1976.

Dr. Benson gives the reader guidelines to a simple medi-
tative technique that has helped millions to cope with
fatigue, anxiety, and stress. Once learned, the relaxation response takes 10 to 20 minutes twice a day, and
can relieve the restlessness and tension that stand between you and a richer, fuller, healthier life.

916. Brown, Barbara. STRESS AND THE ART OF BIOFEEDBACK.
Harper & Row, New York. 1977.

A self-help treatment intended for interested nonprofes-
sionals, this book summarizes the effectiveness of different kinds of biofeedback, which it presents as the
most exciting, far-reaching discovery to emerge from
biomedical research. Clinical uses of biofeedback for
headache, anxiety, tension, insomnia, hypertension,
childbirth, and for hyperactive children are described.
Analyses are presented on which biofeedback—cardiovascular, gastrointestinal, or brainwave—is best for
which person. The book also includes an extensive
bibliography of work in this field.

917. Carrington, Patricia. FREEDOM IN MEDITATION. Anchor
     Press (Doubleday), New York. 1977.

     This book, written by a poet and scientist, covers the
     subject of meditation sensitively and convincingly.

918. Collins, Gary. OVERCOMING ANXIETY. Vision House,
     Santa Ana, Calif. 1975.

919. Cooper, Cary L., and Marshall, Judi. UNDERSTANDING
     EXECUTIVE STRESS. Petrocelli, Princeton, N.J. 1978.

920. De Rosis, Helen. WOMEN AND ANXIETY. Delacorte, New
     York. 1979.

921. Eliot, Robert S.   STRESS AND THE MAJOR CARDIOVASCULAR
     DISORDERS. Futura Publishing, Mount Kisco, N.Y. 1979.

922. Fogarty, Thomas F. COPING WITH STRESS. Claretian
     Publications, Chicago. 1975.

923. Goldberg, Philip. EXECUTIVE HEALTH. McGraw-Hill,
     New York. 1978.

     This collection of excerpts by contemporary experts on
     stress and stress management gives brief but clear
     descriptions of the most common stressors in daily life.
     Approaches to prevention, self-care, and holistic treat-
     ment provide a sound understanding of the stress con-
     cept.

924. Haynes, William D.   STRESS RELATED DISORDERS IN
     POLICEMEN. R&E Research Associates, Palo Alto, Calif.
     1978.

925. Jacobson, Edmund. YOU MUST RELAX. 5th ed. McGraw-
     Hill, New York. 1978.

     Dr. Jacobson, a recognized pioneer in relaxation ther-
     apy, explains simple methods to help relieve nervous
     tension and make life more relaxed and fulfilling.
     This latest edition of a continuing bestseller in-
     structs the reader in effective use of muscular energy
     as a relaxation technique.

926. Keller, W. Phillip. TAMING TENSION. Vantage, New
     York. 1978.

927. Kennedy, Larry W. DOWN WITH ANXIETY. Broadman Press,
     Nashville, Tenn. 1979.

     Dr. Kennedy attempts to help the reader overcome anxi-
     ety through the use of scriptural quotations.

928. Koestenbaum, Peter. MANAGING ANXIETY. Celestial Arts,
     Millbrae, Calif. 1979.

929. Krauss, Hans. BACKACHE, STRESS AND TENSION. Simon &
     Schuster, New York. 1978.

930. Lamott, Kenneth. ESCAPE FROM STRESS, LEARNING RELAXA-
     TION WITH THE RIGHT RESPONSE. Berkley Publishing
     Corporation, New York. 1975.

     The author explains what stress is and answers some of
     the most frequently asked questions on ways to relax.
     The book clearly outlines the causes and effects of
     stress and surveys numerous new techniques for reliev-
     ing and avoiding disorders and diseases related to
     stress. The reader is titillated by relaxation tech-
     niques that promise to lengthen life spans and increase
     talents and abilities.

931. Lecker, Sidney. THE NATURAL WAY TO SUCCESSFUL STRESS
     CONTROL. Grosset & Dunlap, New York. 1978.

932. Levi, Lennart. SOCIETY, STRESS AND DISEASE: THE
     PRODUCTIVE AND REPRODUCTIVE AGE–MALE–FEMALE ROLES AND
     RELATIONSHIPS. Oxford University Press, New York. 1976.

933. Marmorstein, Jerome. THE PSYCHOMETABOLIC BLUES:
     PRACTICAL SOLUTIONS FOR ANXIETY, DEPRESSION, FATIGUE,
     HYPOGLYCEMIA AND RELATED STRESSFUL PROBLEMS. Woodbridge
     Press, Santa Barbara, Calif. 1979.

934. Mason, L. John. GUIDE TO STRESS REDUCTION. Peace
     Press, Culver City, Calif. 1979.

935. May, Rollo. THE MEANING OF ANXIETY. Pocket Books,
     New York. 1979.

936. McQuade, Walter, and Aikman, Ann. STRESS. Bantam,
     New York. 1975.

     Career problems, family hostilities, and the many ten-
     sions of urban living can alter body chemistry. Stress
     plays a major role in almost all chronic diseases, in-
     cluding heart trouble, hypertension, ulcers and other
     digestive ailments, arthritis, cancer, allergy, mi-
     graine, and accident proneness. The reader is advised
     on how to adapt his life to combat the harmful effects
     of stress. This book helps the reader to understand
     what kind of person he is, what stress ailments to ex-
     pect, and what solutions are available, for example,
     biofeedback, hypnosis, psychotherapy, and mysticism.
     The authors have interviewed leading medical special-
     ists and have summarized the research on stress.

937. Mitchell, Laura. SIMPLE RELAXATION. Atheneum, New
     York. 1979.

938. Nideffer, Robert N., and Sharpe, Roger G. HOW TO PUT
     ANXIETY BEHIND YOU. Stein & Day, Briarcliff Manor,
     N.Y. 1978.

     Although a moderate amount of anxiety is said to help
     people reach their peak performance, an overdose may
     cause them to fail consistently. Dr. Nideffer has de-
     vised a training program that enables people to adjust
     to their own stress levels and, thus, perform better at
     their jobs and to enjoy life more. Through case his-
     tories, the authors show how to identify the type of
     stress and anxiety that seems to be controlling one's
     life, which treatments are tailormade to give insight
     into one's own problems, and methods for eliminating
     them. This is a sourcebook for various methods of re-
     lieving stress such as self-hypnosis, biofeedback, TM,
     and yoga.

939. Norfolk, Donald. STRESS FACTOR. Simon & Schuster,
     New York. 1979.

940. Page, Robert C. HOW TO LICK EXECUTIVE STRESS.
     Cornerstone Library, New York. 1977.

941. Pelletier, Kenneth. MIND AS HEALER, MIND AS SLAYER.
     Delacorte, New York. 1977.

     The author maintains that, by relieving stress and
     physical and psychological disease, readers can re-
     formulate their lives and use the time and energy nor-
     mally spent on combating illness to living life as
     fully as possible. The book offers ways to control
     stress and, thus, to prevent stress-related illness.
     One section of the book describes the nature of stress,
     as well as the role of the brain, autonomic nervous
     system, endocrine glands, and the body's immune system.

942. Phillips, Beeman N. SCHOOL STRESS AND ANXIETY. Human
     Science Press, New York. 1978.

943. Phillips, E. L. DAY TO DAY ANXIETY MANAGEMENT. Krieger,
     Huntington, N.Y. 1977.

944. Schwartz, Jack. VOLUNTARY CONTROLS. E. P. Dutton,
     New York. 1978.

     This handbook gives specific, step-by-step instructions
     to obtain powers of self-control developed by the author.
     An important part of this technique is creative medita-
     tion, which embraces reverie, uses of energy, chanting,
     autogenics, and contemplation. The author also shows
     how to activate the chakras, the seven mystical points
     along the spine, each of which has a specific and power-
     ful function.

945. Selye, Hans. THE STRESS OF LIFE. Rev. ed. McGraw-
     Hill, New York. 1978.

     This famous classic has been completely revised and ex-
     panded, with special emphasis on new research findings
     on the subject of stress. How the stress concept was
     first discovered is carefully documented. Advice is
     given on how to observe signs of stress in oneself;
     depression, pounding of the heart, dryness of the throat,
     impulsive behavior, emotional instability, overpowering
     urge to cry or run and hide, inability to concentrate,
     feelings of unreality, weakness or dizziness, loss of
     joie de vivre, nervous ticks, insomnia, sweating, fre-
     quent need to urinate, excessive use of cigarettes,

alcohol, and drugs, a tendency to migraines, nightmares, and accident proneness. The consequences of stress as manifested in diseases of the kidney, heart, and blood vessels are discussed.

946. Sharpe, Robert, and Lewis, David. THE SUCCESS FACTOR. Crown, New York. 1976.

The authors developed a series of response control procedures (RCPs) to enable individuals to advantageously use the principles of behavioral psychology. These RCPs can aid the reader to acquire the habit of success.

947. Sharpe, Robert, and Lewis, David. THRIVE ON STRESS. Warner Books, New York. 1978.

948. Sieber, J. E.; O'Neil, Harold F.; and Tobias, Sigmund. ANXIETY, LEARNING AND INSTRUCTION. Halstead, New York. 1977.

949. Smith, Manual J. KICKING THE FEAR HABIT: USING YOUR AUTOMATIC ORIENTING REFLEX TO UNLEARN YOUR ANXIETIES, FEARS AND PHOBIAS. Dial, New York. 1977.

950. Stuart, Mary E. TO BEND WITHOUT BREAKING: STRESS AND HOW TO DEAL WITH IT. Abingdon, New York. 1977.

951. Tache, Jean; Selye, Hans; and Day, Stacey B., eds. CANCER, STRESS AND DEATH. Plenum, New York. 1979.

This volume represents the outcome of a conference sponsored jointly by the Sloan-Kettering Institute for Cancer Research and the International Institute of Stress. The collection is a classic in the area of cancer and stress, and covers some of the most difficult and complex issues facing the scientific and lay communities.

952. Walker, C. Eugene. LEARN TO RELAX: 13 WAYS TO REDUCE TENSION. Prentice-Hall, Englewood Cliffs, N.J. 1975.

953. Weatherhead, Leslie D. PRESCRIPTION FOR ANXIETY: HOW YOU CAN OVERCOME FEAR AND DESPAIR. Abingdon Press, Nashville, Tenn. 1979.

The aim of this book is to review every known method
of healing through the mind and the spirit. Weatherhead
assesses the place of psychology and religion in the
field of nonphysical healing and passes critical judgment on the methods used to attain health in this field.
The author attempts to ascertain along which lines modern techniques might proceed.

954. Weekes, Claire. PEACE FROM NERVOUS SUFFERING. Bantam,
New York. 1978.

Advice is offered by a doctor to sufferers from nervous
illness. Special fears, loneliness, and depression are
discussed and simple rules for coping are offered: Face
it; Accept it; Let it Float Past; and Let Time Pass.

955. Wheatley, David, ed. STRESS AND THE HEART: INTERACTIONS
OF THE CARDIOVASCULAR SYSTEM, BEHAVIORAL STATE, AND
PSYCHOTROPIC DRUGS. Raven, New York. 1977.

956. Woolfolk, Robert I., and Richardson, Frank C. STRESS,
SANITY, AND SURVIVAL. New American Library, New York.
1979.

NEW AREAS OF HEALTH RESEARCH

Current research into the potential for human self-regulation has increased the use of an ever-growing number of techniques as a means to cope with stress. In the past 10-15 years, voluntary regulation of the involuntary system (autonomic nervous system) has become widely known as a possible achievement.

The focus upon stress as the phenomenon that underlies many illnesses and disabilities led to the impetus to better understand the autonomic nervous system and its control. Heart beat, breathing, muscle tone, and skin temperature are among the host of bodily responses automatically controlled by involuntary responses.

Some societies use techniques which have indicated that control of the autonomic nervous system is possible. But Western medicine and modern science have labeled such mechanisms as quackery and gimmickry. Travelers exposed to Eastern ways prompted clinicians to change their myopic perceptions. Current research in biofeedback techniques, for example, has achieved wide recognition as a legitimate tool for stress reduction.

Awareness of this dangerous predator has encouraged the search for more efficient ways to intercept the damage caused by excessive or prolonged stress. Techniques for meditation and relaxation grow in abundance. A shared common denominator subscribes to the belief that individuals can learn to influence bodily functions to relieve the effects of excessive stress and anxiety.

Biofeedback, the system of self-regulation most often studied scientifically, serves the field as a microcosm for similar techniques, such as meditation, hypnosis, autogenic therapy, and progressive relaxation.

Biofeedback favors an integration of basic psycho-physiological principles and lends itself to measureable precision. Measureable precision has the potential to counteract the belief structures of both physicians and patients who distrust anything that implies a psychological

211

or emotional component. Biofeedback devices help people
to realize that thoughts can control bodily functions
thereby permitting psychological insights to somatic
problems.

The thesis underlying the principle of these techniques is that physiological change is accompanied by a
concurrent change in mental and emotional functioning and
vice versa. For example, the goal of bioenergetic therapy
is the control of muscular movement and breathing. Thermal
feedback devices at the Menninger Clinic have been combined
with other therapy in an active attempt to raise the temperature of the skin. Biorhythm is used by industry and
by individuals in decision planning.

A broad new world for self-regulation is opening up
to examine those important factors that contribute to illness and premature death.

NEW AREAS OF HEALTH RESEARCH

Bioenergetics

957. Becker, Wayne M. ENERGY AND THE LIVING CELL: AN INTRODUCTION TO BIOENERGETICS. Harper & Row, New York. 1977.

958. Broda, E. EVOLUTION OF BIOENERGETIC PROCESSES. Pergamon, New York. 1978.

The central theme of this highly technical book is developed through a discussion of the path from fermentation to photosynthesis and respiration and the relationship of the bioenergetic processes.

959. Heinrich, Bernard. BUMBLEBEE ECONOMICS. Harvard University Press, Cambridge, Mass. 1979.

This different and interesting book uses the bumblebee as a model to explore biological energy costs and pay-offs. The physiological and behavioral bases of the energy economy of the bumblebee are traced to their wider ecological implications.

960. Keleman, Stanley. YOUR BODY SPEAKS ITS MIND. Simon & Schuster, New York. 1975.

This is Keleman's most complete book on understanding the language of our bodies: "We do not have our bodies, we <u>are</u> our bodies." The author writes in a clear and direct manner, allowing the reader to get a good feeling for bioenergetics.

961. Kleiber, Max. FIRE OF LIFE. New ed. Krieger, Huntington, N.Y. 1975.

This introduction to classical bioenergetics has been carefully written so that people with only elementary training in mathematics, physics, and chemistry can understand its contents.

962. Lehninger, Albert L. BIOENERGETICS: THE MOLECULAR BASIS
     OF BIOLOGICAL ENERGY TRANSFORMATIONS. 2nd ed. Benjamin-
     Cummings, Menlo Park, Calif. 1971.

963. Lowen, Alexander. THE BETRAYAL OF THE BODY. Macmillan,
     New York. 1969.

964. Lowen, Alexander. BIOENERGETICS. Penguin, New York.
     1976.

     The author presents an historical review of bioenergetic
     therapy from the works of Wilhelm Reich. In addition,
     the book analyzes a number of common physical disorders
     such as headaches and lower back pain and shows how to
     unlock the tense muscles that can cause these condi-
     tions.

965. Morowitz, Harold J. FOUNDATIONS OF BIOENERGETICS.
     Academic Press, New York. 1978.

     This book, designed for biologists, biochemists, chem-
     ists, and physicists, is a combination of thermal
     physics, biochemistry, ecology, cellular and organismic
     biology. The author's desire is to make the background
     of bioenergetics as clear and unambiguous as possible.

966. Racker, Efraim. A NEW LOOK AT MECHANISMS IN BIO-
     ENERGETICS. Academic Press, New York. 1976.

     This highly technical book is based on the Robbins
     Lectures given by the author at Pomona College in 1973.

967. Szent-Gyorgi, Albert. BIOELECTRONICS. Academic Press,
     New York. 1968.

Biofeedback

968. Baker, Mary; Regenos, Eleanor; Wolf, Stephen; and
Basmajian, John. DEVELOPING STRATEGIES FOR BIOFEEDBACK
APPLICATIONS IN NEUROLOGICALLY HANDICAPPED PATIENTS.
American Physical Therapy Assn., Washington, D.C. 1977.

This pamphlet discusses strategies involving muscle biofeedback applications in the rehabilitation of neurologically handicapped patients. Guidelines in the proper application of electrodes and biofeedback equipment
are presented along with methods of documentation. The
authors offer their training strategies as an initial
guide and stress that uses of biofeedback need to be
explored and documented.

969. Barber, Theodore X. BIOFEEDBACK AND SELF-CONTROL.
Aldine, Chicago. 1975-76.

970. Basmajian, J., ed. BIOFEEDBACK: PRINCIPLES AND PRACTICE
FOR CLINICIANS. Williams & Wilkins, Baltimore. 1979.

This authoritative book on the principles and practices
of biofeedback for the treatment of neurological, psy-
chosomatic, and psychological disturbances is intended
for the clinician. The goal of biofeedback is to make
the patient acquire substantial voluntary control in
cases of stroke, cerebral palsy, and severe recurring
headaches, conditions which in the past have often been
untreatable. Contributors to this volume include experts in the fields of physical therapy, obstetrics,
behavioral science, rehabilitation medicine, internal
medicine, and biofeedback clinicians.

971. Beatty, Jackson, and Heiner, Legewie, eds. BIOFEEDBACK
AND BEHAVIOR. Plenum, New York. 1977.

This volume is the proceedings of a symposium on Biofeedback and Behavior, which was part of the NATO Human
Factors Conference and Symposia Program in Munich in
1976. Seventy scientists from nine nations presented
and discussed recent work on the learned modification
of bodily processes using "biofeedback" procedures.
This record provides the reader with a view of the current state of biofeedback research.

972. Brown, Barbara. STRESS AND THE ART OF BIOFEEDBACK.
     Bantam, New York. 1978.

     The author presents the first comprehensive formulation
     on the use of biofeedback to treat a variety of ill-
     nesses and to relieve conditions related to stress.
     She also outlines biofeedback concepts and discusses the
     role of psychotherapeutic measures. This is a technical
     work which outlines clinical procedures but the inter-
     ested layman should be able to understand the material.

973. Cohen, Daniel. BIOFEEDBACK: A NEW FRONTIER OF THE MIND.
     (Gr. 12, up). Harcourt, Brace, Jovanovich, New York.
     1977.

974. Green, Elmer, and Green, Alyce. BEYOND BIOFEEDBACK.
     Delacorte, New York. 1977.

     This fascinating book attempts to integrate a lifetime
     of scientific work, personal experience, and observa-
     tions relevant to the problem of mind over matter. The
     author's often highly speculative theoretical integra-
     tions present an important challenge.

975. Hartje, Jack C. BIOFEEDBACK: HEALTH WITHOUT DRUGS.
     Hwong Publishing, Los Alamitos, Calif. 1979.

976. Heisel, D. BIOFEEDBACK GUIDE: AFFILIATING WITH
     EXCELLENCE. Gordon & Breach, New York. 1977.

     The author, a professor at the University of Cincinnati,
     is also director of the biofeedback center available to
     students, called Inner Quest. Her book is creatively
     designed to introduce the reader to the software and
     applications of biofeedback.

977. Jencks, Beate. YOUR BODY--BIOFEEDBACK AT ITS BEST.
     Nelson-Hall, Chicago. 1978.

     This practical book can be used for self-training or by
     therapists in physical therapy, psychotherapy, or nurs-
     ing, with individuals or groups. The reader is intro-
     duced to biofeedback and relevant physiological and
     psychological processes. Techniques for coping with
     the stresses of daily life are offered, as well as an

introduction to sensory awareness. Breathing, physical
alignment, physiological processes, and psychological
functioning are also discussed.

978. Karlins, Marvin, and Andrews, Lewis M. BIOFEEDBACK:
TURNING ON THE POWER OF YOUR MIND. Lippincott, New
York. 1972.

979. Lamott, Kenneth. ESCAPE FROM STRESS. Berkley Publ.,
New York. 1975.

Stress of life, stress diseases, meditation, hypnosis,
and biofeedback are all discussed in this excellent
volume on managing stress. The author's concern for his
own survival was the principal motive to write this
book.

980. Mostofsky, D. BEHAVIOR CONTROL AND MODIFICATION OF
PHYSIOLOGICAL ACTIVITY. Prentice-Hall, Englewood
Cliffs, N.J. 1976.

981. Peper, Erik; Ancoli, Sonia; and Quinn, Michele, eds.
MIND-BODY INTEGRATION: ESSENTIAL READINGS IN BIOFEED-
BACK. Plenum, New York. 1978.

This collection of articles on biofeedback is an invaluable tool for the student, professional, or interested
reader. The editors provide overviews, generalizations,
critical analyses, and research studies within a matrix
of knowledge of psychophysiology and instrumentation.
Articles have been chosen from different frameworks,
thus balancing pure and applied areas.

982. Stoyva, Johann, ed. BIOFEEDBACK AND SELF-CONTROL.
Aldine, Chicago. 1979.

983. Yates, A. J. BIOFEEDBACK AND THE MODIFICATION OF
BEHAVIOR. Plenum, New York. 1980.

In this book, the author has attempted to evaluate
critically the large mass of literature which has accumulated in the area of biofeedback over the past 10-
15 years. The literature divides itself into two main
categories--fundamental research studies and therapeutic studies.

984. Alibrandi, Tom. BIORHYTHM. Major Books, Canoga Park, Calif. 1976.

985. Bartel, Pauline. BIORHYTHM: DISCOVERING YOUR NATURAL UPS AND DOWNS. Watts, New York. 1978.

This well-researched and well-written book comes complete with charts and explanations for readers to plot
their rhythms.

986. Blough, Glenn O. DISCOVERING CYCLES (Gr. 3 - 7). New ed. McGraw-Hill, New York, 1978.

987. Dale, Arbie. BIORHYTHM. Pocket Books, New York. 1976.

988. Gale, Mort. BIORHYTHM COMPATIBILITY. Warner Books, New York. 1978.

989. Gedda, Luigi, and Brenci, Gianni. CHRONOGENETICS: THE INHERITANCE OF BIOLOGICAL TIME. Charles C Thomas, Springfield, Ill. 1978.

Chronogenetics is devoted to an exposition of the thesis
that biological time rhythm is hereditary in nature and
"that the mechanism capable of producing, maintaining,
and transmitting it must be sought in the competence of
genetics."

990. Gittelson, Bernard. BIORHYTHM, A PERSONAL SCIENCE. Arco, New York. 1976.

In this clearly-written, easy-to-understand book, the
author discusses the basic tenets of biorhythm and com-
pletely explains methods to chart personal biorhythm
curves and those of the famous and infamous.

991. Handyside, Joann. BIORHYTHMS IN MAN. Dayton Labs, Dayton, Ohio. 1978.

992. Leonard, George. THE SILENT PULSE: A SEARCH FOR THE PERFECT RHYTHM THAT EXISTS IN EACH OF US. Dutton, New York. 1978.

993. Mallardi, Vincent. BIORHYTHMS AND YOUR BEHAVIOR: A PERSONAL DIARY PROGRAM FOR TIME AND LIFE OBJECTIVES. Running Press, Philadelphia. 1978.

This book explores the causes and effects of periodic changes taking place in the human body. Highs and lows, manipulated by varying hormone levels in the bloodstream are recorded along with predictable cycles of minutes, hours, days, weeks, and months. Diary materials are structured for the reader to easily plot past and future tendencies for feelings, stamina, and mental ability.

994. Martin, Lee. THE BIORHYTHM HANDBOOK, WORKBOOK AND FORECASTER. Barnes & Noble, New York. 1978.

995. O'Neill, Barbara, and Phillips, Richard. BIORHYTHMS: HOW TO LIVE WITH YOUR LIFE CYCLES. New American Library, New York. 1976.

This volume demonstrates by explicit graphs the impact of biorhythms in the triumphs and defeats of well-known politicians, entertainers, and sports figures. The authors help the readers to chart their own biorhythms and those of their families, friends, and coworkers. The book shows how to spot "critical days" as well as potentially positive times.

996. Tatai, Kichinosuke. BIORHYTHM FOR HEALTH DESIGN. Japan Publications, New York. 1977.

997. Wernli, Hans J. BIORHYTHM. Cornerstone Library, New York. 1976.

People experience phenomena during their lifetime
consisting of recognized and unrecognized responses that
can affect well-being. One unrecognized pattern of response
that can become harmful is reaction to excessive tension.
Tension (and its emotional companion, anxiety,) is essential to proper mental and physical functioning. However,
an overabundance of tension, manifested in the body by
tight muscles, poor mental coordination, diminished performance, and a general feeling of debilitation can make
people depressed, tired, and prey to disease.

Because homeostasis consists of the proper mix of
tension and relaxation, the state of well-being is often
determined by the way people deal with excessive amounts
of tension and anxiety.

For centuries people have known about the benefits
derived from muscular relaxation by the use of concentra-
tion to relieve tension and anxiety. For example, with
a concentrated mind and relaxed muscles, an athlete can
achieve prize-winning heights of coordination, performance,
and well-being; whereas an athlete with an anxious mind and
a tense body suffers diminished ability and agility regardless of levels of skill.

Techniques to control tension and anxiety have existed
for millenia in every culture. From the rituals of re-
peated prayer and incantation to the patterns of discipline
exhibited by professional athletes, people use techniques
designed to relax and reassure them. Some relaxation
rituals are systematized while others are idiosyncratic in
nature.

Yoga is one of the oldest systematized forms of relaxation. Formerly considered the province of Indian fakirs,
yoga is now being studied and practiced in Western societies.
Western physicians are prescribing yoga to patients with
diabetes, respiratory ailments, digestive complaints, and
obesity. Esoteric phenomena such as brain waves and oxygen
utilization in the blood are examined in response to yoga
techniques. Even some cancer patients are being treated

with yoga (or mind control) techniques, because evidence shows that emotional stress may affect the cause and course of cancer. The philosophy of health manifested by the popularity of yoga recognizes the power of that life force (within mind and emotions) that can either advance or inhibit the course of disease.

Meditation is another form of control over tension and anxiety. Transcendental Meditation (TM) is the most widely known technique used for "getting in touch with oneself". The operational belief is that residing within us lies a balanced center which can be tapped as a guide for the successful resolution of everyday problems. Some changes that can be measured in the body during meditation are a slowing of breath and heart rate, decrease in oxygen consumption, lowering or stabilization of blood pressure, and decrease in skin conductivity.

Variations on this theme are "Relaxation Response", "Clinically Standardized Meditation" and Zen meditation. Regardless of the system that suits the individual, methods exist which promise control over debility common to an excess of tension.

PHILOSOPHIES OF HEALTH

Yoga

998. Acharya, Pundit. BREATH, SLEEP, THE HEART AND LIFE:
THE REVOLUTIONARY HEALTH YOGA OF PUNDIT ACHARYA.
Dawn Horse Press, Clearlake Highlands, Calif. 1975.

This book contains selections from four publications by
the author originally published in the 1950s. The presentation is a combination of practical exercises and
the author's philosophy of life.

999. Ajaya, Swami. YOGA PSYCHOLOGY: A PRACTICAL GUIDE TO
MEDITATION. Rev. ed. Himalayan International Institute, Honesdale, Pa. 1976.

1000. Aurobindo, Sri. BASES OF YOGA. Auromere, Pomona,
Calif. 1979.

1001. Aurobindo, Sri. DICTIONARY OF SRI AUROBINDO'S YOGA.
Auromere, Pomona, Calif. 1979.

1002. Aurobindo, Sri. PRACTICAL GUIDE TO INTEGRAL YOGA.
7th ed. Auromere, Pomona, Calif. 1979.

1003. Bender, Ruth. YOGA EXERCISES FOR EVERY BODY. Ruben
Publications, Avon, Conn. 1975.

This book is a logical, commonsense approach to yoga
exercise. Mrs. Bender is a teacher's teacher, having
trained many yoga teachers over the years.

1004. Brena, Stephen F. YOGA AND MEDICINE. Penguin, New
York. 1973.

This book contends that the average human being has
little control over his/her own mental and physical
health. With this in mind, the author/physician reviews both the medical and yogic concepts of anatomy,

physiology, nutrition, respiration, sexual activity,
pathology, and pain.

1005. Bubba Free John. CONSCIOUS EXERCISE AND THE TRANS-
CENDENTAL SUN. 3rd rev. ed. Dawn Horse Press,
Clearlake Highlands, Calif. 1977.

Conscious exercise is a way of practicing "whole body
happiness." This book describes basic ways to stand,
sit, walk, and breathe with energy and delight; outlines brief and natural routines of calisthenics, hatha
yoga, surya namabar; and includes instructions on the
basic practice of pranayama (control of life-force in
breath) that can be done at random throughout the day.

1006. Carr, Rachel. YOGA FOR ALL AGES. Simon & Schuster,
New York. 1975.

The author presents a six-stage yoga course to enable
the reader to enjoy the benefits of yoga in less than
30 minutes of practice a day. Progressing from simple
movements to the more complex, these exercises aim at
physical conditioning, easing of tensions, and the
promotion of physical, mental, and emotional well-
being.

1007. Carr, Rachel. THE YOGA WAY TO RELEASE TENSION. Barnes
& Noble, New York. 1977.

This book is structured to help the reader relax and
release tension created by daily pressures. On-the-
spot exercises and a selection of 12 yoga exercises
are designed to be done at home. The publication includes deep-breathing exercises on mind control and
body relaxation.

1008. Chinmoy, Sri. YOGA AND SPIRITUAL LIFE. Rev. ed.
Aum Publications, Jamaica, N.Y. 1974.

In this book, the contemporary spiritual, Master Sri
Chinmoy, explains the general philosophy of yoga and
Eastern mysticism. Written in a practical vein, it
offers the newcomer as well as the advanced seeker
a deep understanding of various aspects of the spiritual life. Of particular interest is the section

devoted to questions and answers on the soul and the
inner life.

1009. Christensen, Alice, and Ranklin, David. EASY DOES IT:
YOGA FOR PEOPLE OVER 60. Harper & Row, New York.
1979.

This excellent manual is based on the authors' extensive work with older people. An elderly woman models
for the yoga exercises illustrated in a step-by-step
format. The authors provide background and introductory material on the subject and include a series of
cautions and hints for prudent action.

1010. Couch, Jean. RUNNER'S WORLD YOGA BOOK. World
Publications, Mountain View, Calif. 1979.

1011. Day, Harvey. YOGA FOR THE ATHLETE. New ed. Soccer,
New Rochelle, N.Y. 1976.

1012. Dechanet, J. M. YOGA IN TEN LESSONS. Cornerstone
Press, St. Louis, Mo. 1980.

This introduction to yoga is for those who desire
instruction to yoga theory. Fifty-two exercises with
clear instructions are described, along with information on the therapeutic effects and the attendant
dangers of yoga exercises.

1013. Diskin, Eve. YOGA FOR YOUR LEISURE YEARS. Warner
Books, New York. 1978.

The idea behind this book is: Who's too old for Yoga?
Not you. This step-by-step guide to exercising your
way to renewed flexibility, better health, and joy in
living has no text. Drawings and photographs are clear
and excellent. Miniprograms are presented to choose
from, ranging from the simplest to the most advanced.

1014. Esser, Helen M. FLEXIBILITY AND HEALTH THROUGH YOGA.
Kendall-Hunt, Dubuque, Iowa. 1978.

1015. Hittleman, Richard. RICHARD HITTLEMAN'S THIRTY DAY YOGA
MEDITATION PLAN. Bantam, New York. 1978.

1016. Hittleman, Richard. WEIGHT CONTROL THROUGH YOGA.
Bantam, New York. 1971.

1017. Hittleman, Richard. YOGA: EIGHT STEPS TO HEALTH AND
PEACE. David McKay, New York. 1975.

This well-known author, considered the most prolific
writer on yoga in America today, surveys the different
types of yoga and discusses how the techniques of the
six major systems of yoga can be applied.

1018. Hittleman, Richard. YOGA TWENTY-EIGHT DAY EXERCISE
PLAN. Bantam, New York. 1973.

This book is designed for people who do not have the
time or the inclination for grueling calisthenics.
A four-week, day-by-day exercise program is described
clearly and is well illustrated with photographs.
The author says that, with a minimum of effort, a
maximum effect can be achieved.

1019. Isaacs, Benno, and Kobler, Jay. WHAT IT TAKES TO FEEL
GOOD: THE NICKOLAUS TECHNIQUE. Viking, New York. 1978.

1020. Iyengar, B. K. LIGHT ON YOGA. Rev. ed. Schocken,
New York. 1979.

The author provides detailed instructions on asana
(posture) and pranayama (breathing discipline) including the complete techniques of 200 asanas accompanied
by 592 photographs. These instructions are based on
the author's experience of study and teaching for over
27 years in many parts of the world. The book also
covers bandha and kriya. Some fascinating legends
handed down by practicing yogis and sages are included.

1021. Kriyanada, Swami. FOURTEEN STEPS TO PERFECT JOY: A
HOME-STUDY COURSE IN YOGA. 2nd rev. ed. Ananda,
Nevada City, Calif. 1979.

1022. Leboyer, Frederick. INNER BEAUTY, INNER LIGHT. Knopf,
New York. 1978.

1023. Leuchs, Arne, and Skalka, Patricia. SKI WITH YOGA: CONDITIONING FOR THE MIND AND BODY. Greatlakes Living Press, Chicago. 1976.

1024. Lewis, James R. YOGA FOR COUPLES. Autumn Press, Brookline, Mass. 1979.

1025. Luby, Sue. HATHA YOGA FOR TOTAL HEALTH: HANDBOOK OF PRACTICAL PROGRAMS. Prentice-Hall, Englewood Cliffs, N.J. 1977.

This book is designed to be used by beginning, intermediate, and advanced yoga students. The flow of exercises is planned so that each student can progress to his or her own limit. The publication contains some excellent pictures showing correct and incorrect postures.

1026. Mishra, Rammurti S. YOGA SUTRAS: THE TEXTBOOK OF YOGA PSYCHOLOGY. Doubleday, New York. 1973.

This is a textbook of yoga psychology which describes systematically well-tested methods "to explore the atom of the psyche for the direct perception of its omniscience, omnipotence, and omnipresence."

1027. Moore, Marcia, and Douglas, Mark. YOGA, SCIENCE OF THE SELF. Rev. ed. Arcane Publications, York Harbor, Maine. 1979.

1028. Norton, Suza. YOGA FOR PEOPLE OVER FIFTY: EXERCISE WITHOUT EXHAUSTION. Devin-Adair, Old Greenwich, Conn. 1977.

This book offers a holistic approach for the person over 50 who wants to begin yoga in a realistic manner.

1029. O'Brien, Justin. YOGA AND CHRISTIANITY. Himalayan International Institute. Honesdale, Pa. 1978.

1030. Oki, Masahiro. HEALING YOURSELF THROUGH OKIDA YOGA. Japan Publications, New York. 1977.

1031. Pandit, M. P. DYNAMICS OF YOGA. 3 vols. Auromere, Pomona, Calif. 1979.

1032. Pandit, M. P.   YOGA FOR THE MODERN MAN.   Auromere,
      Pomona, Calif.   1979.

1033. Pandit, Sri.   YOGA OF WORKS.   Auromere, Pomona, Calif.
      1979.

1034. Perkins, Margaret.   YOGA FOR WOMEN'S LIB.   British
      Book Center, Elmsford, N.Y.   1975.

1035. Rama, Swami.   LECTURES ON YOGA.   Rev. 3rd ed.
      Himalayan International Institute, Honesdale, Pa.
      1979.

1036. Rawls, Eugene S.   A HANDBOOK OF YOGA FOR MODERN
      LIVING.   Warner Books, New York.   1978.

      The instructions in this book of yoga are complete.
      You will know the reasons for every movement you make.
      The author includes detailed practice schedules.

1037. Rawls, Eugene, and Diskin, Eve.   JOY OF LIFE THROUGH
      YOGA.   Warner Books, New York.   1976.

      This informative book describes the purpose of yoga
      and the different types--Hatha, Raja, Bhakti, Karma,
      and Mantra.   The idea of self-improvement is empha-
      sized and suffering--its existence, its cause, and
      its cure--is confronted head-on.

1038. Ross, Karen.   THE NEW MANUAL OF YOGA.   Arco, New York.
      1977.

1039. Shandler, Nina, and Shandler, Michael.   YOGA FOR
      PREGNANCY AND BIRTH: A GUIDE FOR EXPECTANT PARENTS.
      Schocken, New York.   1979.

      This excellent book for expectant parents is concerned
      with the presence of God within expectant mothers and
      fathers and within their babies.   The authors respon-
      sibly delineate the systems and methods of yoga while
      reminding the reader of the spirit behind yoga.

1040. Shankaranayanan, S.   TEN GREAT COSMIC POWERS.
      Auromere, Pomona, Calif.   1979.

1041. Sharma, Pandit-Shi.   YOGA AND SEX.   Cornerstone
      Library, New York.   1975.

1042. Venkatesanda, Swami. YOGA. Strawberry Hill Press, San Francisco. 1980.

1043. Werner, Karel. YOGA AND INDIAN PHILOSOPHY. South Asia Books, Columbia, Mo. 1979.

This book is based on material which has been used by the author in academic courses as well as in classes of adult education. The author has made it as readable as possible for those members of the general public who are interested in the theme while, at the same time, preserving the book's standard as a reliable introduction to Indian philosophical teachings and the teachings of yoga.

1044. White, John, ed. KUNDALINI, EVOLUTION AND ENLIGHTEN- MENT. Doubleday, New York. 1979.

1045. Yesudian, Sebarajan. SELF-RELIANCE THROUGH YOGA. 3rd ed. Allen Unwin, Winchester, Mass. 1979.

1046. Young, Frank R. YOGA SECRETS FOR EXTRAORDINARY HEALTH AND LONG LIFE. Barnes & Noble, New York. 1977.

1047. Zebroff, Kareen. THE ABC OF YOGA. Arco, New York. 1979.

This self-teaching manual contains simple step-by-step yoga exercises for beginners. Introductory information covers diet, meditation, breath control, and specific do's and don'ts to get the most from yoga.

1048. Berry, Thomas. RELIGIONS OF INDIA: SCHOOL EDITION. Glencoe, Encino, Calif. 1971.

1049. Carr, Rachel E. BE A FROG, A BIRD OR A TREE: RACHEL CARR'S CREATIVE YOGA EXERCISES FOR CHILDREN (Gr. 4 - 7). Doubleday, New York. 1973.

For all children who want to be healthy and strong, this large, attractive paperback has appealing and charming illustrations, drawings, and photographs of both animals and children. The exercises are a simulation of positions one sees in the animal and plant kingdoms.

1050. Cheki-Haney, Erene, and Richards, Ruth. YOGA FOR CHILDREN. Bobbs-Merrill, Indianapolis, Ind. 1973.

1051. Diskin, Eve. YOGA FOR CHILDREN (Gr. 7 - 11). Arco, New York. 1977.

Designed by a famous author and teacher, this guide to yoga is for children to use by themselves.

1052. Glovach, Linda. THE LITTLE WITCH'S BOOK OF YOGA (Gr. 2 - 5). Prentice-Hall, Englewood Cliffs, N.J. 1979.

1053. Kuvalayananda, Swami. POPULAR YOGA ASANAS (Gr. 9, up). C. E. Tuttle, Rutland, Vermont. 1972.

1054. Landau, Elaine. YOGA FOR YOU (Gr. 7, up). Messner, New York. 1977.

1055. Luchs, Esther. YOGA FOR YOUNG CHILDREN. Paulist Press, New York. 1977.

1056. Marshall, Lyn. YOGA FOR YOUR CHILDREN. Schocken, New York. 1979.

Designed for both parents and children, this large-format paperback offers fun sessions for achieving the most perfect form of body movement and improvement. Positions described and illustrated include the

triangle, body roll, push up, sit up, lie down, leg
pull, side bend, squat, coil, cobra, and cat.

1057. Richards, Ruth, and Abrams, Joy. LET'S DO YOGA (Gr. 2
- 5). Holt, Reinholt & Winston, New York. 1975.

The authors' intention is to encourage young children
in the practice of physical fitness. This book is well
illustrated with a clear explanation of asanas (postures).

1058. Turner, Alice K. YOGA FOR BEGINNERS (Gr. 5, up).
Watts, New York. 1973.

Just as the title indicates.

1059. Zebroff, Kareen, and Zebroff, Peter. YOGA FOR KIDS
(Gr. 7, up). Sterling Publishing, New York. 1978.

All of the 32 exercises, from Warm-Up and easy Keep-Fit
poses such as the cobra, the camel, the stork, on
through the Intermediate Lotus and Advanced Hatha yoga
poses, are shown in 130 photos accompanied by easy-to-
read instructions.

1060. Adam, Michael. WANDERING IN EDEN: THREE WAYS IN THE EAST WITHIN US. Knopf, New York. 1976.

1061. Bancroft, Ann. ZEN, DIRECT POINTING TO REALITY. Thames Hudson, New York. 1979.

1062. Benoit, Hubert. SUPREME DOCTRINE: PSYCHOLOGICAL STUDIES IN ZEN THOUGHT. Penguin, New York. 1968.

1063. Brandon, David. ZEN IN THE ART OF HELPING. Dell, New York. 1978.

The book contemplates the phenomenon of "helping" and examines people who help for a living, e.g., nurses, doctors, social workers, and teachers. The author attempts to show that this process should be consider- ed a way of living and being rather than be viewed as a particular job or career. He objects strongly to the aridity of much that passes for professionaliza- tion particularly in the helping profession.

1064. Franck, Frederick, ed. ZEN AND ZEN CLASSICS. (Selec- tions from R. H. Blyth.) Random House, New York. 1978.

1065. Fromm, Erich; Suzuki, D. T.; and DiMartino, R. ZEN BUDDHISM AND PSYCHOANALYSIS. Harper & Row, New York. 1970.

This classic book resulted from a workshop on Zen Buddhism and Psychoanalysis which was held at the National University of Mexico in 1972. The volume consists of lectures delivered at the conference by world renowned D. T. Suzuki, Fromm's paper on Psycho- analysis and Zen Buddhism, and Richard DiMartino's paper "Human Situation and Zen Buddhism."

1066. Hoover, Thomas. ZEN CULTURE. Random House, New York. 1978.

This is a concise history of the development of Zen in Japan, why it still permeates Japanese life, and why it has touched a nerve in the West. The influence of Zen

on art, architecture, literature, flower arrangement,
design, archery, and swordsmanship is explained.

1067. Humphreys, Christmas. ZEN: A WAY OF LIFE. Little,
Brown and Co., Boston. 1971.

1068. Humphreys, Christmas. ZEN COMES WEST: THE PRESENT AND
FUTURE OF ZEN BUDDHISM IN WESTERN SOCIETY. 2nd ed.
Rowman, Totowa, N.J. 1977.

Christmas Humphreys, no stranger to the subject of Zen
Buddhism, has worked tirelessly with Alan Watts and
D. T. Suzuki in efforts to bring Eastern and Western
philosophies together. Discussion covers Zen Buddhism
and methods of Zen instruction. Humphreys concludes
with a summary of the situation to date on the practice of Zen and the effect of Zen study on the Europe
of tomorrow.

1069. Izutzu, Toshihiko. TOWARD A PHILOSOPHY OF ZEN BUDDHISM.
Great Eastern, Boulder, Colo. 1978.

1070. Kapleau, Roshi P. ZEN: DAWN IN THE WEST. Doubleday,
New York. 1979.

The author is an American who, while living in Japan
years ago, met three outstanding Zen masters. He now
heads a Zen Center in Rochester, N. Y. His book offers
advice on how to find a Zen teacher, the role of moral-
ity, and social responsibility in dealing with issues
like abortion, suicide, euthanasia, and war.

1071. Kennett, Roshi J. ZEN IS ETERNAL LIFE. 2nd ed. Dharma
Publications, Emeryville, Calif. 1976.

1072. Low, Albert. ZEN AND CREATIVE MANAGEMENT. Doubleday,
New York. 1976.

The author shows how the practice and discipline of Zen
can help avoid the state of servomechanism which is
prevalent in industry today. In review of this work,
Marshall MacLuhan states, "In planning today, the problem is how to head off and control effects by antici-
pating them. In the electric age, effects come before
causes, as in the case of the instant replay ... Men

have always tended to be the servants to their technologies. Zen and Creative Management suggests means of
by-passing this fate."

1073. Maezumi, Hakuyu, and Glassman, Bernard T. FOUNDATIONS
OF PRACTICE. Vol. I, Zen Writing Series. Center
Publications, Los Angeles. 1976.

1074. Maezumi, Hakuyu, and Glassman, Bernard T. BODY, BREATH
AND MIND. Vol. II, Zen Writing Series. Center
Publications, Los Angeles. 1976.

1075. Maezumi, Hakuyu, and Glassman, Bernard T. THE HAZY
MOON OF ENLIGHTENMENT. Vol III, Zen Writing Series.
Center Publications, Los Angeles. 1978.

This book attempts to lead the reader along the path to
enlightenment. First, the author examines enlightenment itself, then he explores the ways in which delu-
sion obscures or hinders enlightenment. Finally, he
discusses in detail the eight awarenesses of the enlightened person, Shakyamuni Buddha's last teaching,
and provides a map of the enlightened life.

1076. Maezumi, Hakuyu, and Loori, John D. THE WAY OF EVERY-
DAY LIFE. Center Publications, Los Angeles. 1978.

The authors replace spiritual and psychological para-
phenalia with gentle unassuming words, color photographs, and a Zen master's text, to beckon the reader
to look more realistically at life.

1077. Powell, Robert. ZEN AND REALITY: AN APPROACH TO SANITY
AND HAPPINESS ON A NONSECTARIAN BASIS. Penguin,
New York. 1977.

A very clearly written, well-referenced book on Zen
wherein the author discusses Krishnanurti, Zen, and
the reasons and need for Buddhism.

1078. Ross, Nancy W., ed. THREE WAYS OF ASIAN WISDOM:
HINDUISM, BUDDHISM, ZEN. Touchstone Books, New York.
1978.

1079. Sato, Koji. THE ZEN LIFE. New ed. Weatherhill, New
York. 1977.

This photo-essay depicts life at Empuku-ji Monastery.
It discusses the tradition and creativity of Zen,
entering a Zen monastery, the discipline of zazen
(seated meditation), Zen food, marriage, education,
and other facets of daily living.

1080. Sekida, Katsuki. ZEN TRAINING: METHODS AND PHILOSOPHY.
Weatherhill, New York. 1975.

The author, who has practiced and studied Zen for an
uninterrupted period of 60 years, writes for the serious Zen student. According to Mr. Sekida, the unques-
tioned basis of any serious practice of Zen is zazen,
the exercise in which the student sits and learns to
control his mind and body. Therefore, a substantial
part of this book is devoted to describing the per-
formances and effects of zazen. The book also describes the psychology of consciousness, of cognition,
and of samadhi of Kenshio.

1081. Sekiguchi, Shindri. ZEN: A MANUAL FOR WESTERNERS.
Japan Publications, Tokyo and New York. 1970.

This book is a guide for those who know little or
nothing about Zen Buddhism. The volume is for Westerners who are unaware of the traditional and historical
setting of the Buddhist faith. The author sketches the
basic doctrines of Buddhism, relates them to Zen meditation, and then details the mental approach and physical
effects of zazen.

1082. Stone, Justin F. ZEN MEDITATION. (A BROAD VIEW.)
Sun Publications, Albuquerque, N. Mex. 1975.

1083. Suzuki, D. T. THE ESSENTIALS OF ZEN BUDDHISM. Greenwood, Westport, Conn. 1973.

These primers are just what their titles indicate: an
introduction to Zen for beginners and a manual en-
abling the reader to pursue further studies in Zen.
The author (1870 - 1966), universally considered the
greatest authority in the world on Zen Buddhism, was

also the pioneer teacher of Buddhist philosophy out-
side Japan.

1084. Suzuki, D. T.   THE AWAKENING OF ZEN.   Great Eastern,
Boulder, Colo.   1980.

1085. Thien-An, Thieh.   BUDDHISM AND ZEN IN VIETNAM: IN
RELATION TO THE DEVELOPMENT IN ASIA.   C. E. Tuttle,
Rutland, Vt.   1975.

1086. Thien-An, Thieh.   ZEN PHILOSOPHY, ZEN PRACTICE.   Dharma
Publications, Emeryville, Calif.   1975.

1087. Watts, Alan.   NATURE, MAN AND WOMAN.   Random House,
New York.   1970.

Watts discusses man's place in the natural world and
the present-day alienation and hostility to nature so
common in modern men and women.   Writing as a poet and
a philosopher, Watts believes that the love of a man
and a woman is a sacramental means of overcoming es-
trangement from life.

1088. Watts, Alan.   THE WAY OF ZEN.   Random House, New York.
1974.

1089. Watts, Alan.   THREE.   Pantheon Books, New York.   1977.

1090. Wu, John C.   THE GOLDEN AGE OF ZEN.   Paragon, New York.
1975.

Meditation

1091. Allport, Gordon W. WAITING FOR THE LORD: 33 MEDITA-
TIONS ON GOD AND MAN. Macmillan, New York. 1978.

This book of meditations compiled by a professor of
psychology guides the reader to resources in the Bible.
These meditations are suggestive and not doctrinaire,
and are designed to allay persistent problems the
thoughtful reader will face.

1092. Ames, Louise A. MEDITATIONS FOR YOUTH. Beta Book,
San Diego, Calif. 1979.

1093. Bjorge, James R. AND HEAVEN AND NATURE SINGS.
Concordia Publishing, St. Louis, Mo. 1977.

1094. Boyd, Malcolm. AM I RUNNING WITH YOU, GOD? Doubleday,
New York. 1977.

This book of short stories and sensitive poems reveals
the author's conflicting feelings of fear of and con-
tentment with God.

1095. Bryant, Al. DAILY MEDITATIONS WITH F. B. MEYER. Word
Books, Waco, Texas. 1979.

1096. Butts, Mary. LO, THE WINTER IS PAST. Vantage, New
York. 1978.

1097. Casey, Lawrence B. THE HEART REMEMBERS, TOO. Paulist
Press, New York. 1977.

This collection of articles reflects the author's life,
work, and faith. The book discusses Bishop Casey's
participation in the Second Vatican Council, but deals
primarily with family life, changing seasons, and personal friends.

1098. Cavert, Walter D. REMEMBER NOW. Abingdon, Nashville,
Tenn. 1979.

1099. Chapman, J. Wilbur. SECRET OF A HAPPY DAY. Baker Book
House, Grand Rapids, Mich. 1979.

Chapman offers 30 daily readings as meditations for Christians, as ways of maintaining one's spirit and calm by prayer in the midst of "modern" living.

1100. Clark, Wayne C.   GOD IS MY STRENGTH.   Judson Press, Valley Forge, Pa.   1977.

1101. Colman, Henry, ed.   DIVINE MEDITATIONS.   Yale University Press, New Haven, Conn.   1979.

1102. Conners, Kenneth W.   LORD, HAVE YOU GOT A MINUTE? Judson Press, Valley Forge, Pa.   1979.

This creatively illustrated book is about the pains, joys, and growth experienced by Christians of all ages and denominations.

1103. Emmons, Helen B.   THE MATURE HEART.   New ed. Abingdon, Nashville, Tenn.   1977.

This volume explores ways to live in harmony with the conditions around us and with the Spirit of God within us.   The meditations are arranged in a progressive order of topics to be read consecutively or at random by using the subject index.

1104. Gordon, Arthur.   TOUCH OF WONDER.   Revell, Old Tappan, N.J.   1974.

A simple book that conveys a sense of gratitude for the endless free gifts that life offers.   The author invites the reader to fall in love with life and thereby set in motion the mysterious dynamics that will cause life to love in return.

1105. Hallesby, O.   GOD'S WORD FOR TODAY: A DAILY DEVOTIONAL FOR THE WHOLE YEAR.   Augsburg, Minneapolis.   1979.

1106. Havner, Vance.   HOPE THOU IN GOD.   Revell, Old Tappan, N.J.   1978.

This book of 52 short sermons contains the author's personal experiences and shows his profound feelings for the Bible.

1107. Hill, Jeanne. DAILY BREATH. Word Books, Waco, Texas.
      1978.

      A wife, mother, registered nurse, and professional
      writer offers the reader many practical inspirations
      as ways to lighten the load and add deeper meaning to
      a burdened life.

1108. Hulme, William E. LET THE SPIRIT IN: PRACTICING
      CHRISTIAN DEVOTIONAL MEDITATION. Abingdon, Nashville,
      Tenn. 1979.

      The author explains his ambivalent feelings about the
      relation of daily devotions to spiritual development.
      The book discusses the complementary nature of man's
      analytical and rational abilities and his capacity for
      the intuitive, the artistic, and the sensuously imag-
      inative, and how these differing capacities form a
      balance in human life.

1109. Johnson, David. GUIDELINES: THOUGHTS ON CHRISTIAN
      LIVING. Wallace-Homestead, Des Moines, Ia. 1978.

1110. Jones, E. Stanley. HOW TO BE A TRANSFORMED PERSON.
      Abingdon, Nashville, Tenn. 1978.

      This book attempts to relate transformation to man's
      spiritual growth and development through the gentle
      fusion of literary and spiritual sensibilities. The
      author writes for Christians interested in meditation
      and Oriental philosophy.

1111. Kagawa, Toyohiko. MEDITATIONS. Greenwood, Westport,
      Conn. 1979.

1112. Keen, Sam. BEGINNINGS WITHOUT END. Harper & Row,
      New York. 1977.

1113. Keshavadas, Sadguru S. GAYATRI, THE HIGHEST
      MEDITATION. Vantage, New York. 1979.

1114. Koyama, Kosuke. FIFTY MEDITATIONS. Orbis Books,
      Maryknoll, N.Y. 1979.

Koyama's beautiful, earthy book of meditations represents a synthesis of Oriental thought and Christianity.

1115. Lauterbach, William A. THROUGH CLOUD AND SUNSHINE.
Concordia Publishing, St. Louis, Mo. 1979.

These 41 calm devotions attempt to inspire us to face
with God the vagaries of everyday living. Each devo-
tion is based on a particular scripture in achievement
of a natural balance.

1116. McKenna, Marylou. SERENITY BOOK. Rawson Wade, New
York. 1978.

1117. Malinski, Miecryslaw. OUR DAILY BREAD. Seabury Press,
New York. 1979.

This beautifully written book of daily meditations
offers practical counsel on ways to enrich Christian
living.

1118. Mow, Anna B. SPRINGS OF LOVE. Brethern Press, Elgin,
Ill. 1979.

1119. Mullen, Tom. BIRTHDAYS, HOLIDAYS AND OTHER DISASTERS.
Word Books, Waco, Texas. 1978.

This book attempts to convey the humorous side of everyday events which, when taken too seriously, can sometimes prove disastrous. The author's humorous, anec-
dotal musings on becoming a teenager to taking long
motor trips with children are designed to help keep
problems and achievements in perspective.

1120. Murphy, Elspeth C. CHALKDUST: PRAYER MEDITATIONS FOR
A TEACHER. Baker Book House, Grand Rapids, Mich. 1978.

1121. Oates, Wayne E. NURTURING SILENCE IN A NOISY HEART.
Doubleday, New York. 1979.

This book discusses silence in man's daily life, the
need for quiet moments, and offers instruction on what
the author means by "down-to-earth centering."

1122. Perry, Oberlin W., Sr., and Perry, Chandler R. INSPIRATIONAL READINGS. Vantage, New York. 1978.

1123. Roach, Fred. LET'S TALK: IDEAS TO TRIGGER FAMILY CONVERSATION. Revell, Old Tappan, N.J. 1977.

1124. Roberts, William P. AT THE DOOR KNOCKING. Pflaum-Standard, Fairfield, N.J. 1975.

1125. Rockness, Miriam H. KEEP THESE THINGS, PONDER THEM IN YOUR HEART, REFLECTIONS OF A MOTHER. Doubleday, New York. 1979.

This is a book of reflections on the frustrations, questions, fears, and joys unique to mothering. The author writes about everyday experiences and offers understanding and support for every woman facing the responsibilities and joys of motherhood.

1126. Rothacker, Reg V. PRECIOUS JEWELS. Vantage, New York. 1979.

1127. Russell, Marjorie H. HANDBOOK OF CHRISTIAN MEDITATION. Devin-Adair, Old Greenwich, Conn. 1978.

This easy-to-understand, practical handbook offers a variety of meditations for Christians who wish to enrich their spiritual life. The author is an internationally known lecturer, teacher, and counselor.

1128. Shrader, Elizabeth H., and Hand, Katherine. MEDITATIONS ON ANCIENT WISDOM. Creative Press, Claremont, Calif. 1977.

1129. Sibley, Celestine. SMALL BLESSINGS. Doubleday, New York. 1977.

This delightfully simple book discusses topics ranging from windowsills to weeds to authentic tales of folk-lore and how these things can enhance daily life.

1130. Taliaferro, Margaret. DO YOU EVER HAVE QUESTIONS LIKE THESE? Doubleday, New York. 1979.

1131. Ten Boom, Corrie.   EACH NEW DAY.   Revell, Old Tappan,
      N.J.   1977.

1132. Tengbom, Mildred, and Tengbom, Luverne.   FILL MY CUP,
      LORD: MEDITATIONS ON WORD PICTURES IN THE NEW
      TESTAMENT.   Augsburg, Minneapolis.   1979.

      Thirty-three key Greek words in the New Testament form
      the basis of the enriching meditations found in this
      volume.   Based on the authors' travels and research,
      facets of meaning are opened and imaginative pictures
      are recovered aiding the reader in a sense of history,
      science, and religion.

1133. Tilman, Klemans.   MEDITATIONS IN DEPTH.   Paulist Press,
      New York.   1979.

1134. Vuilleumier, Marion.   MEDITATIONS BY THE SEA.   Abingdon
      Press, Nashville, Tenn.   1980.

1135. Ward, Benedicta.   PRAYERS AND MEDITATIONS OF ST.
      ANSELM.   Penguin, New York.   1979.

SELF-HEALTH

In spite of technological advances in medical care,
the single most significant factor in the maintenance of
health or recovery from illness is the body's natural
healing functions. By a variety of medical techniques,
sophisticated medical care can assist the healing powers
of the body and interrupt the course of a disease. Spec-
tacular as medicine is in certain instances, the human
organism, nonetheless, is unexcelled in its ability to
resist illness and heal injuries. The goal of the pro-
ponents of self-health is to help reinforce the attributes
of natural healing resources.

Although some Americans may view the phenomenon of
natural healing and self-health as radical and mystical,
many cultures have been using natural approaches to health
for centuries. Medical practice aims for the quick cure;
natural healing takes a slower, organic approach. Herbs,
for example, have been used for centuries for the relief
of pain and to assist healing. According to empiric observation, herbs enhance healing processes, strengthen
and rejuvenate the body, and provide the blood with beneficial effects. Although many of our modern-day medications
are synthetics, they are derived from living plants and
fungi. Cross-cultural studies of literature and behavior
reveal a dependence on herbal remedies that have been handed
down from one generation to another. Ancient Egyptians,
Chinese, Persians, Romans, Greeks, Babylonians, and Hebrews
have documented their use of herbs as remedial agents. The
American Indians have found products in the forest and in
the field to alleviate ills.

Medicine and science have reappraised their indifferent
attitude toward folk medicine and are now examining world-
wide herbal and other remedies common to earlier epochs
of history. Large drug firms are exploring tropical jungles
for roots, leaves, barks, and seeds.

Coupled with the search for old remedies is a new
emphasis on the "holistic" approach which contrasts sharply
with the mechanistic view dominating much of medicine today.
Holism is an ancient term for a modern theory: Living

nature is more than the sum of its parts. For example,
to treat a human being, a physician should not only know
the interrelations of organs and tissues, but should also
account for the person's surrounding environment and
understand his/her emotional and spiritual essence.

Holistic health care begins with the belief that all
aspects of a person affects the cause and outcome of illness and strongly emphasizes the emotional and mental
factors in health and illness. The mechanistic view sees
the person as parts of a machine which are to be studied
and treated separately.

A promising factor in a holistic approach is the focus
on individual responsibility for prevention of illness
which can effectively control problems of modern health
care.

SELF-HEALTH

General

1136. Airola, Paavo. HOW TO GET WELL. Health Plus Publications, Phoenix, Ariz. 1974.

Written by a world-famous authority on nutrition and natural healing, this practical manual describes common ailments and tells the reader what to do about them. The author discusses nutritional and biological therapies which are directed at correcting the underlying causes of disease, strengthening the person's resistance to disease, and creating the most favorable conditions for the body's own healing processes. This book is an excellent source for professionals and informed laymen.

1137. Ardell, Donald B. HIGH LEVEL WELLNESS. Bantam Books, New York. 1979.

This well-known guidebook to optimal health and well-being describes ways to shape a positive **lifestyle for** a longer life. The author provides **self-tests** to determine present levels of wellness and offers revitalizing diets and other health-enhancing practices. The reader is introduced to several holistic health centers where wellness, not medicine, is prescribed for healthy and ill alike.

1138. Austin, Glenn. PARENTS' MEDICAL MANUAL. Prentice-Hall, Englewood Cliffs, N.J. 1978.

1139. Bernhard, Yetta. SELF CARE. Celestial Arts, Millbrae, Calif. 1975.

Much of this book is devoted to transcriptions of the author's work with patients, which dramatically supports her claim that "the practice of self-care is the process by and through which self-respect, self-worth, and self-liking are developed."

1140. Blackie, Margery C. THE PATIENT NOT THE CURE: THE
CHALLENGE OF HOMEOPATHY. Woodbridge Press, Santa
Barbara, Calif. 1978.

In this well-written book, the author, physician to the
Queen of England and honorary consulting physician to
the Royal London Homeopathic Hospital, discusses the
concepts of homeopathy, materia medica, homeopathic
teaching, and 20th century practitioners.

1141. Bricklin, Mark. THE PRACTICAL ENCYCLOPEDIA OF NATURAL
HEALING. Rodale Press, Emmaus, Pa. 1976.

The author, executive editor of Prevention magazine,
has written the first complete book that brings together the most popular natural healing techniques,
from acupuncture to herbal medicine to yoga therapy.
The book provides a variety of information on treating
health problems without drugs.

1142. Galton, Lawrence. HOW LONG WILL I LIVE? AND 434 OTHER
QUESTIONS YOUR DOCTOR DOESN'T HAVE TIME TO ANSWER AND
YOU CAN'T AFFORD TO ASK. Macmillan, New York. 1976.

1143. Gardner, A. Ward. GOOD HOUSEKEEPING DICTIONARY OF
SYMPTOMS. Grosset & Dunlap, New York. 1978.

1144. Gomez, Joan. DICTIONARY OF SYMPTOMS. Stein & Day,
Briarcliff Manor, N.Y. 1977.

This is a quick-and-easy reference book written by a
British physician who is the mother of ten children.
The book is indexed for easy emergency use and has
separate sections on children, men, and women. It
answers hundreds of questions, such as the difference
between a heart attack and acute indigestion, how to
tell a tension headache from high blood pressure, how
serious diseases of childhood can be prevented, and
what some of the danger signals are as a woman gets
older. A glossary of medical terms is included.

1145. Hammond, Sally. WE ARE ALL HEALERS. Ballantine Books,
New York. 1974.

This solid, objective report on psychic healing today

discusses laying-on-of-hands, faith healing, absentee
healing, and presents interviews with these famous
healers: Olga Worall, Harry Edwards, Rolling Thunder,
Gordon Turner, Lawrence LeShan, and Rev. Alex Holmes.

1146. Horowitz, Steve, and Offen, Neil. CALLING DR.
HOROWITZ. BJ Publication Group, New York. 1978.

1147. Johnson, T. C. DOCTOR! WHAT YOU SHOULD KNOW ABOUT
HEALTH CARE BEFORE YOU CALL A PHYSICIAN. McGraw-Hill,
New York. 1975.

This guide to the health care market is based on the
author's experience in dealing with those seeking
health care and medical attention for emergencies,
heart and lung diseases, cancer, women's health problems, infections, and gastrointestinal disorders. The
book summarizes significant health information in these
areas and provides guidance where choices may be
important. It addresses such questions as: What kind
of health care do you need? How to find it? How to
check the credentials of a doctor or a hospital? What
new information is worth knowing and what old information is still important?

1148. Katz, Robert S. MEDICAL TESTS YOU CAN DO YOURSELF.
Sterling Publishing, New York. 1978.

1149. Lipkin, Mack. STRAIGHT TALK ABOUT YOUR HEALTH CARE.
Harper & Row, New York. 1977.

1150. Miller, Benjamin, and Galton, Lawrence. COMPLETE
MEDICAL GUIDE. 4th ed. Simon & Schuster, New York.
1978.

This extensively illustrated guide includes the latest
and most authoritative findings used in medical practice and for the care of all parts of the body. The
style is simple, informative, and friendly. Topics
range from health in childhood, youth, maturity, and
old age, to reducing diets, pregnancy, danger signals
of heart trouble, cancer, and hypertension, as well as
preparation for marriage and sex. A comprehensive
dictionary of medical terms is included.

1151. Miller, Jonathan. THE BODY IN QUESTION. Random House,
      New York. 1979.

1152. Ornstein, Dolph. MEDICINE TODAY, HEALING TOMORROW.
      Celestial Arts, Millbrae, Calif. 1976.

      This book is about the exciting new concept of health
      care based on improved nutrition, an awareness of sex-
      uality, and the prevention of disease. The author also
      offers an excellent discussion on herbs.

1153. Pomerantz, Virginia, and Schultz, Dodi. MOTHERS AND
      FATHERS MEDICAL ENCYCLOPEDIA. Rev. ed. New American
      Library, New York. 1978.

1154. Rosenberg, M. M. ENCYCLOPEDIA OF MEDICAL SELF-HELP:
      MEDICINE FOR THE MILLIONS. Publishers Agency, Glen-
      dale, Md. 1979.

1155. Rosenfeld, Isadore. THE COMPLETE MEDICAL EXAM. Simon
      & Schuster, New York. 1978.

      Good medical care depends on the free flow of informa-
      tion between doctor and patient--in both directions.
      The purpose of this book is to enhance this communica-
      tion by explaining and presenting information neces-
      sary to understand what happens during a medical
      examination and why.

1156. Rothenberg, Robert E. WHAT EVERY PATIENT WANTS TO
      KNOW. New American Library, New York. 1975.

1157. Samuels, Mike, and Bennett, Hal. BE WELL. Random
      House, New York. 1975.

      A book that satisfies the general reader's quest for a
      common-sense guide to health, it clearly and simply
      states how people can take responsibility for being
      healthy. Since most people now realize that present
      day attitudes and behavior promote our own "dis-ease,"
      it follows, the authors claim, that we have the power
      within us to change our responses to life thereby
      preventing the emergence of "dis-ease."

1158. Samuels, Mike, and Bennett, Hal.   THE WELL BODY BOOK.
Random House, New York.   1978.

This comprehensive home medical handbook written by
physicians describes in excellent detail how to do a
complete physical exam, how to diagnose common diseases, how to practice preventive medicine, and how to
get the most from your doctor.   The authors include
step-by-step illustrations and an annotated bibliography.

1159. Shealy, C. Norman.   90 DAYS TO SELF-HEALTH.   Dial
Press, New York.   1977.

Biogenics, a word meaning origin of life, is an elabo-
rate system of mental exercises designed to help regu-
late the body's functions.   The author outlines the
system developed in working with over 1300 patients
and in conducting a number of clinical research projects, combining biofeedback, autogenic training, auto-
suggestion, Gestalt psychology, and psychosynthesis.
This practical, enjoyable workbook provides a three-
month program for enhancing one's health.

1160. Steincrohn, Peter J.   ASK DR. STEINCROHN: WHAT YOU
ALWAYS WANTED TO ASK YOUR DOCTOR AND DIDN'T.   Acropolis
Books, Washington, D.C.   1979.

Dr. Steincrohn maintains that good health depends on
what you know, and this book attempts to fill the void
left by uncommunicative visits to your doctor.   The
book covers every topic from weight loss, how to find
the best physician, how to handle a dying relative,
how to tell if you have cancer, to alcoholism, smoking,
jogging, mammography, and snoring.

1161. Tawshunsky, Ben.   EFFECTIVE REMEDIES FOR COMMON
AILMENTS.   Exposition Press, Hicksville, N.Y.   1977.

1162. Taylor, Robert B.   DR. TAYLOR'S SELF-HELP MEDICAL GUIDE.
New American Library, New York.   1978.

1163. Thosteson, George.   THE EVERYDAY MEDICAL HANDBOOK.
Fawcett, New York.   1977.

1164. Vickery, Donald M., and Fries, James. TAKE CARE OF
YOURSELF: A CONSUMER'S GUIDE TO MEDICAL CARE. Addison-
Wesley, Reading, Mass. 1976.

This useful handbook provides self-diagnosis charts
and home treatment information for 68 common medical
problems. These easy-to-read charts clearly indicate
when to use home treatment and when to call the doctor.
The authors offer practical advice on choosing the
right doctor, the office visit, a home pharmacy, and
the right medical facility.

1165. Zinman, Joseph Aaron. SECRETS OF HEALTH THAT MANY
DOCTORS AND DENTISTS MAY NOT KNOW. Exposition Press,
Hicksville, N.Y. 1977.

1166. Beckett, Sarah. HERBS FOR PROSTATE AND BLADDER
TROUBLE. British Book Center, Elmsford, N.Y. 1978.

The author provides a line drawing and an alphabeti-
cally arranged discussion of 25 herbs. The three
major herbs indicated to ease prostate distress are
buchu leaves, uva-ursi, and saw palmetto. The book
includes some general information and a therapeutic
guide.

1167. Ceres. HERBS FOR FIRST-AID AND MINOR AILMENTS.
British Book Center, Elmsford, N.Y. 1978.

The first in a series known as Everybody's Home Herbal,
this handy reference describes and illustrates 20
herbs that are easy to obtain and are considered
valuable first-aid for treating minor ailments. The
author often quotes the well-known herbalists, Culpeper and Gerard.

1168. Coon, Nelson. USING PLANTS FOR HEALING. Rodale
Press, Emmaus, Pa. 1979.

This useful guide shows the reader how to take advantage of the remarkable healing qualities of over 250
American plants. Readers can find relief from over
50 diseases and discomforts with the help of easy-to-
find and often very familiar plants. The author, an
octogenarian, considered an authority on medicinal
plants in the U.S., describes the healing qualities
of such familiar spices and foods as cloves, honey,
molasses, mustard, olive oil, sodium bicarbonate,
burned toast, vinegar, and yeast.

1169. Culpeper, Nicholas. COMPLETE HERBAL. Rev. ed. (1st
published by Foulsham & Co., London, 1730.) Wehman,
Cedar Knolls, N.J. 1960.

This book offers a comprehensive description of many
herbs and their medicinal properties. It includes
color pictures of herbs, places to find them, and directions for use. The author cites a list of diseases
and their herbal remedies. Although this book is over
250 years old, it has retained its popularity.

1170. Dawson, Adele. HEALTH, HAPPINESS AND THE PURSUIT OF HERBS. Stephen Greene Press, Brattleboro, Vt. 1979.

1171. De-Bairacli-Levy, Juliette. COMMON HERBS FOR NATURAL HEALTH. Schocken, New York. 1974.

The author is a combination farmer, botanist, and herbalist who has learned about herbal medicine from Bedouins, Spanish gypsies, and American and Mexican Indians. The book describes how to make medicine from common herbs, to use herbs for cosmetic purposes, and to prepare food. The book contains 97 illustrations of different herbal plants.

1172. Gorden, Lesley. GREEN MAGIC: FLOWERS, PLANTS AND HERBS IN LORE AND LEGEND. Viking, New York. 1977.

1173. Kaaiakamanu, D. M. and Akina, J. K. HAWAIIAN HERBS OF MEDICINAL VALUE. C. E. Tuttle, Rutland, Vt. 1972.

1174. Kloss, Jethro. BACK TO EDEN. 5th ed. Woodbridge Press, Santa Barbara, Calif. 1975.

This popular herbal is a potpourri of material on natural cures, suggested remedies for specific diseases and information on preparation of foods.

1175. Latorre, Dolores L. COOKING AND CURING WITH HERBS IN MEXICO. Encino Press, St. Austin, Texas. 1977.

1176. Lavine, Sigmund A. WONDERS OF HERBS (Gr. 5, up). Dodd, Mead, New York. 1976.

1177. Leek, Sybil. SYBIL LEEK'S BOOK OF HERBS. T. Nelson, Nashville, Tenn. 1973.

This book examines mythology of herbs, the history of their use, their culinary, cosmetic, and medicinal value, as well as the lives of several herbalists.

1178. Lucas, Richard. SECRETS OF THE CHINESE HERBALISTS. Prentice-Hall, Englewood Cliffs, N.J. 1977.

The secrets of Chinese herbs are fully discussed and both medicinal information and folklore are offered.

The bulk of the book is devoted to an analysis of the remedial effects of specific herbs for a variety of ailments. The author writes clearly and has a thorough knowledge of his material.

1179. Muir, Ada. HEALING HERBS OF THE ZODIAC. Llewellyn Publications, St. Paul, Minn. 1975.

This is a study of herbs pertaining to each of the 12 signs of the zodiac. Ms. Muir describes how to combine herbs respective of planetary laws and the active principals within each herb.

1180. Rose, Jeanne. JEANNE ROSE'S HERBAL BODY BOOK. Grosset & Dunlap, New York. 1976.

This excellent herbal clearly explains recipes for cosmetic herbal preparation. About one-quarter of the book is devoted to plant descriptions and the author includes a cosmetic glossary and suggestions on where to buy herbs.

1181. Stuart, Malcolm, ed. THE ENCYCLOPEDIA OF HERBS AND HERBALISM. Grosset & Dunlap, New York. 1979.

1182. Thomson, William A. HERBS THAT HEAL. Scribner, New York. 1977.

1183. Weslager, C. A. MAGIC MEDICINES OF THE INDIANS. Middle Atlantic Press, Wallingford, Pa. 1973.

This is a well-written comprehensive survey of the herbal treatments and folklore of the Indians of New Jersey, Pennsylvania, Delaware, and Maryland. It includes information on plants and trees and specific cures.

1184. Bach, Edward. THE BACH FLOWER REMEDIES. Keats, New Canaan, Conn. 1979.

The author, an English physician, feels that sickness and disease are primarily due to some disharmony within the sufferer himself and not to physical causes. The author has extracted 38 medicinal remedies from wildflowers, bushes, and trees for various physical ailments. These remedies are prescribed according to the sufferer's state of mind--moods of fear, worry, anger, or depression--and not directly to the physical complaint. They can be safely used by anyone.

1185. Clark, Linda. HOW TO IMPROVE YOUR HEALTH. Keats, New Canaan, Conn. 1979.

1186. Collier, Richard B. PLENEURETHIC: WAY OF LIFE, SYSTEM OF THERAPEUTICS. Exposition Press, Hicksville, N.Y. 1979.

1187. Gaedwag, E., ed. INNER BALANCE: THE POWER OF HOLISTIC HEALING. Prentice-Hall, Englewood Cliffs, N.J. 1979.

As an alternative option to expensive drugs and traditional methods of treating illness, Inner Balance shows people how to use techniques to control their health. With contributions written by notable leaders in the medical and spiritual community such as Hans Selye, Marcus Bach, and Elisabeth Kubler-Ross, the book describes the proper stress-free physical and mental environment for fighting and preventing disease. The authors explain the use of meditation, imagery, biofeedback, and other "self-direction" methods.

1188. Halpern, Ruben, and Halpern, Joshua. THE ART AND PRACTICE OF HOLISTIC HEALING. Ross-Back Roads, Berkeley, Calif. 1979.

1189. Johnson, Michael L. HOLISTIC TECHNOLOGY. Libra, Roslyn Heights, N.Y. 1977.

The author explores a variety of holistic technologies

and their interconnections with cultural situations. This excellent resource discusses design and community, the interface of art and technology, expanded cybernetics, evolution and consciousness, among other topics.

1190. Kulvinskas, Viktoras. THE NEW AGE DIRECTORY, Survival Foundation, Inc., Haddam, Conn. 1978.

This directory provides a unique and excellent resource for anyone interested in alternative therapies, associated organizations, co-ops, whole food suppliers, and the like.

1191. LaPatra, Jack. HEALING: THE COMING REVOLUTION IN HOLISTIC MEDICINE. McGraw-Hill, New York. 1978.

This book examines the possibility of simple health care for body, mind, and spirit simultaneously. The author's personal research and observations are interwoven with reports from others practicing this kind of healing.

1192. Oyle, Irving. THE NEW AMERICAN MEDICINE SHOW: DISCOVERING THE HEALING CONNECTION. Unity Press, Santa Cruz, Calif. 1979.

1193. Pelletier, Kenneth R., ed. HOLISTIC MEDICINE: FROM PATHOLOGY TO OPTIMUM HEALTH. Delacorte, New York. 1977.

This book is intended as a bridge between the public and the physician. Written by leading experts in teaching on stress, the contributors discuss what holistic medicine is and how it is changing medical care. The principle is that a sound mind in a sound body has a direct bearing on longevity, pathology, and disease prevention.

1194. Sobel, David. WAYS OF HEALTH: HOLISTIC APPROACHES TO ANCIENT AND CONTEMPORARY MEDICINE. Harcourt Brace, New York. 1979.

1195. Thompson, Carroll J. HOLISTIC HEALING. Anthelion Press, Corte Madera, Calif. 1979.

1196. Walker, Morton. TOTAL HEALTH; THE HOLISTIC ALTERNATIVE
TO TRADITIONAL MEDICINE. Everest House, New York.
1979.

In this unique book Dr. Walker has assembled and as-
sessed the basic components of the "holistic medicine"
movement currently sweeping the country. The author
examines the utility of many different methods dealing
with the unnatural health problems in today's civilization.

1197. Wood, Robert H. THE USE OF MASSAGE IN FACILITATING
HOLISTIC HEALTH. Charles C Thomas, Springfield, Ill.
1979.

AUTHOR INDEX

A

Abbo, F.E., 47
Abrams, J., 1057
Acharya, P., 998
Adam, M., 1060
Adams, B., 335
Adams, G., 93
Addeo, E.G., 275
Aero, R., 48
Agee, J., 546
Agran, L., 749
Agrawal, K.C., 868
Agress, C.M., 208
Aikman, A., 936
Airola, P., 376, 720, 1136
Ajaya, S., 999
Akina, J.K., 1173
Ald, R., 278
Alibrandi, T., 192, 984
Allen, E., 209
Allen, J., 210
Allen, Richard, 834
Allen, Robert, 835
Allen, W.A., 795
Allport, G.W., 1091
Alpert, J., 759
Altamura, M.V., 98
Altman, I., 664
Altman, N., 501
Amada, G., 836
Amary, I.B., 837
American Heart Assn., 760
Ames, L.A., 1092
Amit, Z., 122
Ancoli, S., 981
Anderson, A., 544
Anderson, B., 211

Anderson, D.J., 123
Anderson, J., 380, 503
Anderson, L., 579
Anderson, R.A., 913
Anderson, S., 840
Anderson, W.F., 94
Andrews, L.M., 978
Angel-Levy, P., 805
Angerman, G., 795
Annarino, A.A., 212
Anthony, E.J., 888
Anton, T., 684
Appisson, B., 78
Archer, J., 180, 692
Ardell, D.B., 1137
Arena, J.M., 402
Arieti, S., 889
Arlin, M.T., 377
Arms, S., 586
Arneil, S., 336
Arnold, O., 1
Arnow, E.E., 378
Ashdown-Sharp, P., 587
Ashford, N.A., 685
Ashley, R., 379
Astrand, P.O., 213
Atchley, R.C., 95
Aurobindo, S., 1000, 1001,
                   1002
Austin, G., 1138
Axon, W.E., 502

B

Bach, E., 1184
Bach-y-Rita, P., 564
Baden, M., 139
Bailey, C., 214

257